HEMOSTASIS &
THROMBOSIS
A CONCEPTUAL APPROACH

JACK HIRSH, M.D.
Professor of Pathology and Medicine
Chief of Service—Hematology
McMaster University Medical Centre
Hamilton, Ontario, Canada

ELIZABETH A. BRAIN, M.D.
Learning Resources Editor
Health Sciences Education
McMaster University Medical Centre
Hamilton, Ontario, Canada

Illustrated by
KNUD C. SKOV, McMaster University

Churchill Livingstone New York, Edinburgh and London 1979

CHURCHILL LIVINGSTONE
Medical Division of Longman Inc.

Distributed in the United Kingdom by Churchill Livingstone,
23 Ravelston Terrace, Edinburgh EH4 3TL and by associated
companies, branches and representatives throughout the world.

First published by McMaster University 1976
First revision published by Churchill Livingstone 1979
ISBN 0 443 08056 9

Library of Congress Cataloging in Publication Data
Hirsh, Jack, 1935—
    Hemostasis and Thrombosis: a conceptual approach.

    Bibliography: p.
    1. Blood—Coagulation, Disorders of. 2. Hemostasis. 3. Thromboembolism.
    4. Hemorrhagic diseases. I. Brain, Elizabeth A., 1933—   joint author.
    II. Skov, Knud C., joint author. III. Title. [DNLM: 1. Hemostasis. 2. Thrombosis.
    WH310 H489c]
    RC647. C55H57   1979   616.1'5   78-21850
    ISBN 0-443-08056-9

Cover Designed by JAHNUS VIZON

HEMOSTASIS &
THROMBOSIS
A CONCEPTUAL APPROACH

Table of Contents

Preface

This printed, visually oriented text has been prepared for use within the self-instructional M.D. programme at McMaster University. It is not a textbook in that it does not cover all aspects of the field and you will need to turn to other references for details of disease classification and laboratory procedures. It is however a book which has been developed from a series of slide-tape shows on "The Bleeding Disorders" by Dr. Jack Hirsh and produced by McMaster University. The book stands on its own, but also complements the slide-tape shows. We have used this essentially "audio-visual" approach to simplify the major pathophysiological concepts involved in the understanding of normal and abnormal hemostatic processes and thromboembolism. An appreciation of these concepts is necessary for the assessment, clinical and laboratory diagnosis and management of patients with bleeding disorders or suffering from thromboembolic disease. This material is therefore suitable for use by medical students, medical residents, trainees in hematology, medical laboratory technologists, and for the continuing education of internists and hematologists. You will notice that each chapter ends with some self assessment questions. We have purposely not given you the answers to these questions. They are all to be found within the substance of the text. If you find that you cannot answer them to your satisfaction, may we suggest that you review the text, and if you are still having problems, consult your teachers.

Chapter 1

An Introduction to Normal & Abnormal Hemostatic Mechanisms

Function of Hemostasis

1. Prevention of blood loss from intact vessels.

2. Arrest of bleeding from injured vessels.

The function of the normal hemostatic mechanism is to prevent blood loss from intact vessels and to stop excessive bleeding from severed vessels.

Factors Controlling Hemostasis

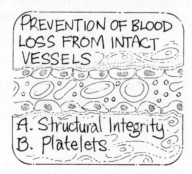

PREVENTION OF BLOOD LOSS FROM INTACT VESSELS

A. Structural Integrity
B. Platelets

The mechanism by which blood is prevented from being shed from intact vessels is uncertain, but the structural integrity of the vessels and the presence of normal platelets is necessary for this function.

ARREST OF BLEEDING FOLLOWING TRAUMA

A. Reaction of blood Vessels.
B. Formation of Platelet Plug.
C. Blood Coagulation.

Arrest of bleeding following trauma is controlled by three interrelated factors. These three factors are the reaction of blood vessels to injury, the formation of the platelet plug at the site of injury, and the coagulation of blood.

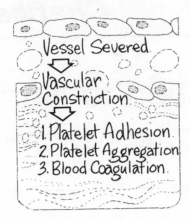

This is a simplified scheme of the normal hemostatic mechanism. When a blood vessel is severed the vessel constricts, blood is shed, and the processes of platelet adhesion, platelet aggregation, and blood coagulation are initiated.

Vessel Constriction

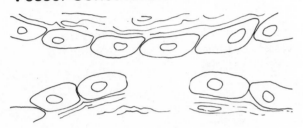

Vascular constriction is transient lasting less than one minute. The mechanism of vascular constriction is uncertain but could be contributed to by a local contractile response to injury or by humoral substances either released from platelets or generated as a result of activation of blood coagulation.

Formation of Unstable Platelet Plug

STEP 1 : Platelet Adhesion
Endothelial Cells
Red Blood Cell
Platelet
Collagen
Release of ADP
ADP

Platelets adhere to the subendothelial connective tissue and to the basement membrane, release adenosine diphosphate, and then aggregate under the influence of the adenosine diphosphate to form an unstable platelet plug.

STEP 2 : Platelet Aggregation

Unstable
Hemostatic
Plug

The formation of the unstable platelet plug by the platelet aggregates takes place within seconds of vessel injury.

Stabilization of Plug with Fibrin

STEP 3 : Blood Coagulation

Platelet Plug
Consolidation

Fibrin Formation

The unstable platelet plug is stabilized after a few minutes, when fibrin, which is the final product of the blood coagulation process, consolidates the plug rendering it stable. The fibrin component of the hemostatic plug gradually increases in amount as the platelets undergo autolysis, so that after 24-48 hours the hemostatic plug is transformed into fibrin.

Fibrinolysis

STEP 4: Fibrinolysis

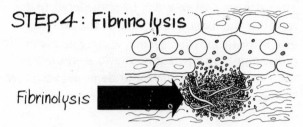

Fibrinolysis

Fibrin is then gradually digested by the fibrinolytic enzyme system and the defect in the wall
of the vessel is covered with endothelium.

Interaction of Platelet Factors &
Coagulation

1. Vaso-active substance released when Platelet comes into contact with Collagen.

2. Blood coagulation is accelerated by platelet aggregation through Phospholipid.

3. Thrombin causes Platelets to release A.D.P.

The processes of platelet adhesion and aggregation, blood coagulation and vessel constriction are closely interrelated. Thus, vasoactive
substances which cause vessel constriction are
released when platelets come in contact with
subendothelial connective tissue. Platelet
aggregation accelerates the process of blood
coagulation by making phospholipid available.
Thrombin, an enzyme which is produced during
blood coagulation, causes platelets to release
adenosine diphosphate.

Blood Coagulation

The process of blood coagulation occurs as a series of complex steps which terminate in the formation of a fibrin clot.
Blood coagulation occurs either by activation of the intrinsic
pathway, which is a relatively slow process, or the activation
of the extrinsic pathway, which is a much faster process.

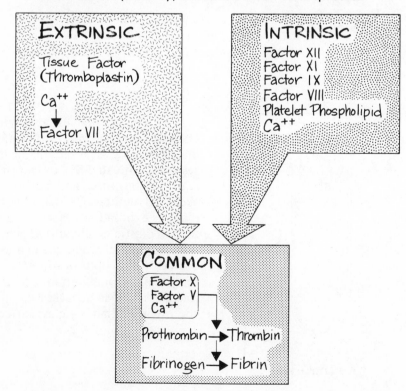

EXTRINSIC

Tissue Factor
(Thromboplastin)

Ca^{++}

Factor VII

INTRINSIC

Factor XII
Factor XI
Factor IX
Factor VIII
Platelet Phospholipid
Ca^{++}

COMMON

Factor X
Factor V
Ca^{++}

Prothrombin → Thrombin

Fibrinogen → Fibrin

Intrinsic Clotting System

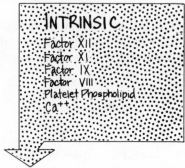

The intrinsic pathway will be considered first as this is the most important of the two systems. The intrinsic clotting system is activated when blood comes in contact with a foreign surface, such as a prosthetic device or damaged vessel wall. This can be demonstrated experimentally both in vivo & in vitro.

In Vivo

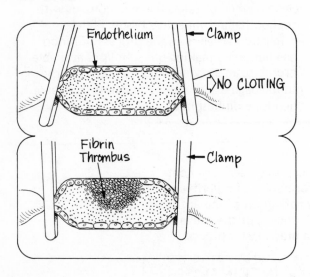

Activation of coagulation in vivo can be induced by minor vessel injury. If a segment of a vein is carefully isolated and clamped at both ends, the blood will remain fluid for days; this is shown in the upper diagram. On the other hand, if the endothelium of the vein is damaged, clotting will occur, because exposure of the subendothelial tissues to blood initiates clotting by activating Factor XII (ie. — the Intrinsic Pathway) and possibly also by making tissue thromboplastin available, & thus activating the extrinsic pathway also.

In Vitro

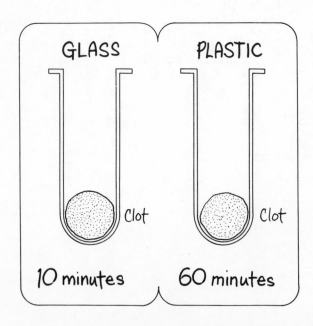

This experiment can also be performed in vitro. If the blood is drawn carefully and placed into a glass tube, the intrinsic clotting system is activated by contact of Factor XII with the glass tube, and clotting occurs in about 10 minutes. On the other hand, if the blood is exposed to a non-wettable surface such as plastic or siliconized glass, activation is less rapid and blood coagulation may be delayed for an hour or more. It seems, therefore, that the non-wettable, plastic or siliconized glass surface behaves more like normal endothelium than the glass surface.

6

Activation of Intrinsic Pathway

Activation of the intrinsic system is shown here. The coagulation factors circulate in the form of inactive precursors, some of these are pro-enzymes or zymogens and some of these are co-factors. Each zymogen is converted into an active form (the enzyme) and in turn activates the next clotting factor in the sequence. This concept has been likened to a cascade or water-fall.

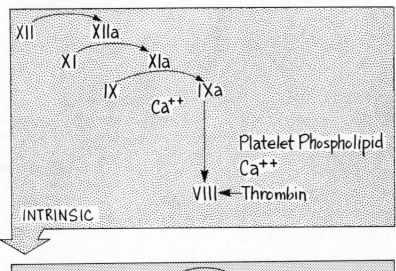

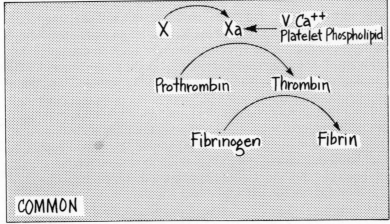

Clotting by the intrinsic pathway begins with activation of factor XII by its exposure to a foreign surface. This surface is glass in the in vitro test systems used, and is probably collagen when the intrinsic system is activated in vivo.

The activated factor XII in turn activates factor XI to form a contact product. This step is calcium independent. The contact product in the presence of calcium, platelet phospholipid, factor IX, and factor VIII, activates factor X.

Factor VIII is a co-factor which is required for the activation of factor X by activated factor IX. The activation of factor X by the factor VIII complex is accelerated by the presence of thrombin and by the availability of platelet phospholipid.

Role of Factor XII

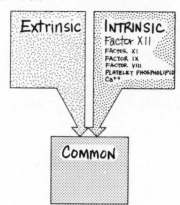

The mechanism of Factor XII activation has recently been clarified.

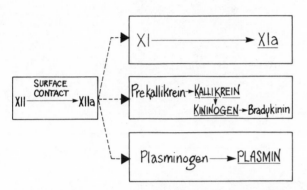

Factor XII is partly activated by contact with a foreign surface in a non-proteolytic step, that is, the molecule is not cleaved. This form of activated XII is a relatively weak activator of a number of reactions, including activation of factor XI, activation of prekallikrein and activation of plasminogen activator.

The products of these reactions, particularly kallikrein, feedback to produce cleavage of the Factor XII molecule to Factor XII fragments. These Factor XII fragments are much more powerful activators of the subsequent steps, that is the conversion of Factor XI to XIa, prekallikrein to kallikrein and plasminogen to plasmin (the fibrinolytic enzyme system).

All 3 of these proteolytic enzymes are capable of cleaving Factor XII to form Factor XIIa fragments which are much more effective in inducing the formation of activated Factor XI, of kallikrein and of plasmin. Kallikrein also converts kininogen to bradykinin and it appears that kininogen also plays a role in Factor XII activation.

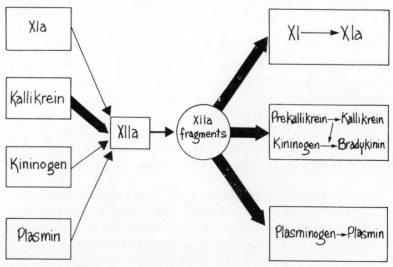

Support for the role of prekallikrein and kininogen in Factor XII activation is provided by studies of families with deficiencies in prekallikrein (also known as Fletcher Factor after the first family with this defect) and kininogen (also known as Fitzgerald Factor after the first family). In both instances there is impaired surface activation of Factor XII with a corresponding prolongation of the in vitro coagulation tests.

Relationship of Coagulation to other Homeostatic Mechanisms

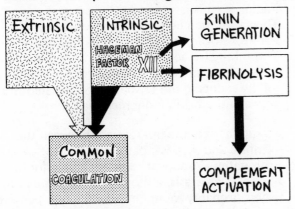

Thus the activation of Factor XII and the associated zymogens discussed above form an important link between a number of homeostatic functions. These include blood coagulation through Factor XII and XI, inflammation through the kinins, fibrinolysis through plasmin and complement activation through plasmin also.

Extrinsic Clotting System

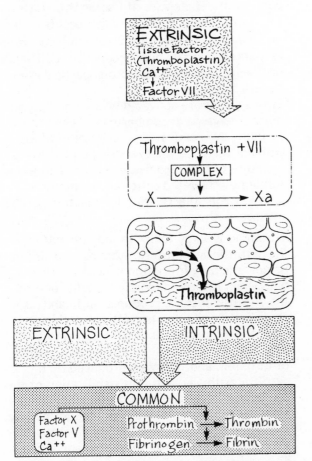

Consider now the extrinsic pathway. When extracts of various tissue such as brain or lung (known as thromboplastin) are added to blood, a number of early time-consuming steps in the intrinsic clotting system are bypassed, and coagulation occurs more rapidly as a result of the activation of the extrinsic system.

Thromboplastin forms a complex with Factor VII which in the presence of calcium, activates Factor X.

The extrinsic pathway is stimulated in vivo by exposure of blood to damaged endothelium or to extravascular tissues, both of which have been shown to have tissue thromboplastin material.

The steps in the activation of the intrinsic and extrinsic pathway lead to a common point at the activation of Factor X, and beyond this point blood coagulation continues along a common pathway.

Interaction of Extrinsic & Intrinsic Pathways

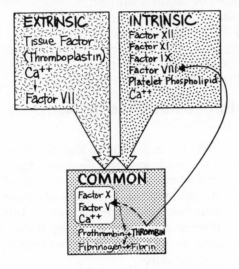

The intrinsic and extrinsic pathways interact in vivo, thus, small amounts of thrombin are formed early following stimulation of the extrinsic pathway when blood comes in contact with extravascular connective tissue, and this in turn accelerates clotting by the intrinsic pathway activating Factor VIII and activating Factor V (this is shown by the arrows). Thrombin then converts the soluble protein fibrinogen into an insoluble fibrin gel. Thrombin also activates Factor XIII which in the presence of calcium, stabilizes the fibrin gel, by inducing the formation of co-valent bonds between the fibrin monomer chains.

To summarize, the interactions between the extrinsic and intrinsic pathways in vivo: —
Both pathways appear to be necessary for normal hemostasis, although the intrinsic pathway is probably more important. Thus, patients with deficiencies of the intrinsic clotting factors have hemorrhagic disorders, as do patients with congenital deficiencies of Factor VII. However, the hemorrhagic disorder which occurs with deficiency of this extrinsic clotting factor is not as marked as that which occurs with deficiencies of the intrinsic clotting factors, particularly Factors VIII and IX.
Both systems are activated when blood passes out of the vascular compartment. The intrinsic pathway is activated by contact of blood with collagen and the extrinsic pathway by exposure of blood to tissue extract. Thrombin formed by the rapid action of the extrinsic pathway acts to accelerate the reactions of the intrinsic pathway.

1. Both Systems needed for Hemostasis.

2. Both Systems activated when vessel damaged.

3. Thrombin accelerates Intrinsic Pathway.

The Role of Thrombin

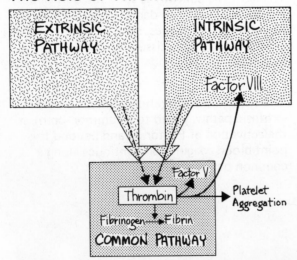

Thrombin is a key factor in the interaction of the extrinsic and intrinsic systems, and also in hemostatic plug formation in general. Thrombin, which is formed rapidly by activation of the extrinsic system, produces fibrin and also feeds back to accelerate clotting, by the intrinsic pathway through activation of Factors VIII and V. It is probable that only small amounts of thrombin and fibrin are produced by the extrinsic pathway, and that stabilization of the hemostatic plug is delayed until sufficient amounts of thrombin and fibrin are formed by activation of the intrinsic pathway. Thrombin also stimulates platelets to release adenosine diphosphate and, therefore, to aggregate. Thus, this enzyme plays a very important role in hemostasis.

Pathogensis of Defective Hemostasis

| Vascular Defects |
| Thrombocytopenia |
| Platelet Function Defects |
| Coagulation Defects |
| Fibrinolysis |

It follows from the discussion on the physiology of hemo-stasis that abnormal bleeding may be caused by: 1) A defect in blood vessels, a so-called vascular defect; 2) By a deficiency in platelets — this is known as thrombocytopenia; 3) By abnormalities of platelet function, — this is known as thrombocytopathia; 4) By defects in blood coagulation and 5) By excessive fibrinolytic activity.

Vascular Defects

- Inherited
- Acquired

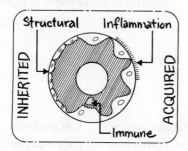

Defects in blood vessels may be inherited or acquired.

The inherited defects are due to structural abnormalities in the vessels themselves and the acquired abnormalities may be due to inflammatory disorders or immune disorders affecting the blood vessels. The acquired disorders occur much more commonly in medical practice.

Platelet Abnormalities

Thrombocytopenia
- Inherited
- Acquired

Thrombocytopenia or a deficiency in the number of circulating platelets may also be inherited or acquired and again, the acquired form occurs much more commonly.

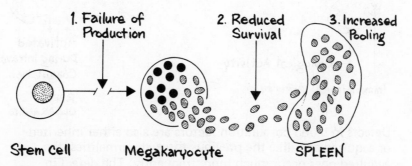

Thrombocytopenia may occur as a result of failure of platelet production, as a result of excessive platelet destruction, or a result of pooling of platelets in an enlarged spleen. Normally, approximately 20% of platelets are pooled at any one time in the human spleen, but if the spleen becomes very large, up to 90% of these platelets may be pooled in the spleen.

Platelet Function Defects

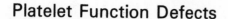

1. Failure of Platelets to Adhere
Failure to Release A.D.P.

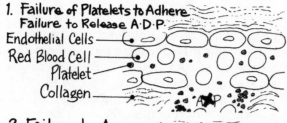

Endothelial Cells
Red Blood Cell
Platelet
Collagen

2. Failure to Aggregate

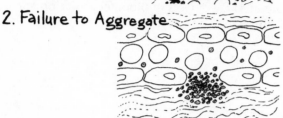

3. Failure to make Phospholipid Available

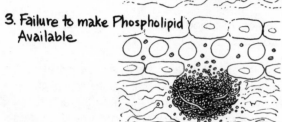

Inherited platelet function abnormalities have been recognized for a number of years, but it is only in recent times that the much more commonly occurring acquired platelet function defects have been appreciated in clinical practice. These abnormalities in platelet function may be caused

by failure of platelets to adhere to exposed subendothelium;

by failure of platelets to release adenosine diphosphate;

by failure of platelets to aggregate with adenosine diphosphate or

by failure of platelets to make phospholipid available, this defect leading to delayed thrombin generation & hence fibrin formation around the platelet aggregate.

Coagulation Defects

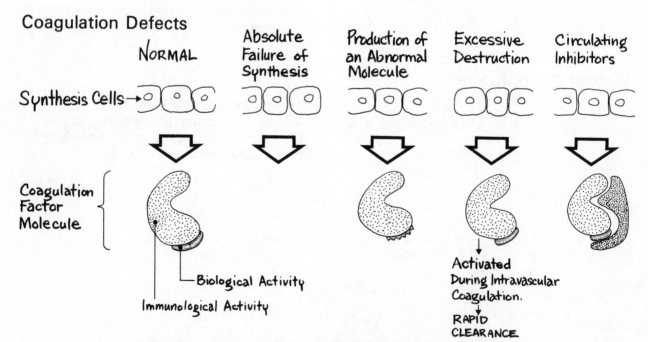

| | NORMAL | Absolute Failure of Synthesis | Production of an Abnormal Molecule | Excessive Destruction | Circulating Inhibitors |

Synthesis Cells →

Coagulation Factor Molecule

Biological Activity
Immunological Activity

Activated During Intravascular Coagulation.
→ RAPID CLEARANCE

Defects in blood coagulation factors are also either inherited or acquired and, like the previous three abnormalities, the acquired ones occur much more frequently. The defect in blood coagulation may be due to an absolute failure of synthesis of coagulation factors, to the production of an abnormal coagulation factor molecule, to excessive destruction of coagulation factors, during intravascular coagulation or to the presence of circulating inhibitors which are usually antibodies to the blood coagulation factors.

Excessive Fibrinolysis

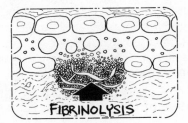

Excessive fibrinolytic activity usually arises as a result of sudden release of tissue activator into the blood stream and may be contributed to by a failure to inactivate this activator by the liver.

Dangers of Abnormal Bleeding

Dangers of
Abnormal Bleeding

1. Blood loss – Anoxia
   – Hypovolemic
     Circulatory Failure
2. Pressure on Vital
   Structures
3. Chronic Anemia
4. Joint & Muscle Deformities

Finally, what are the clinical problems produced by abnormal bleeding? Firstly, morbidity may be produced from blood loss alone, resulting in acute anemia and hence acute anoxia or hypovolemic circulatory failure; secondly, abnormal bleeding may produce pressure on vital structures such as the pharynx resulting in asphyxia, the brain, resulting in severe neurological deficit, or blood vessels, producing gangrene; thirdly, chronic blood loss may result in chronic anemia, and finally bleeding into joints and muscles may lead to contractures and deformities, as a result of the healing process and laying down of fibrous tissue in muscles and joints.

Self Evaluation for Chapter 1

1. How do platelets participate in the normal hemostatic mechanism?
   They participate in the formation of the _____

   _____ by:
   (1)_____
   (2)_____
   (3)_____
   (4)_____

2. Although the extrinsic pathway is intact in patients with hemophilia they bleed abnormally. Why?

3. What are the roles of thrombin in normal hemostatis
   (1)_____
   (2)_____
   (3)_____
   (4)_____

4. What is the stimulus to activation of the intrinsic clotting pathway?
   (1) In vivo _____
   (2) In vitro_____

5. What is the stimulus to activation of the extrinsic clotting pathway?

6. What are the mechanisms of thrombocytopenia
   (1) _____
   (2) _____
   (3) _____

7. What are the mechanisms by which a coagulation factor deficiency can be produced?
   (1) _____
   (2) _____
   (3) _____
   (4) _____

Chapter 2

Clinical Diagnosis of Bleeding Disorders

Definitions

1. Petechiae
2. Purpura
3. Ecchymosis, bruise
4. Hematoma
5. Hemarthrosis
6. Hematuria

These are some of the terms used to describe the more common manifestations of bleeding seen in clinical practice.

Petechiae

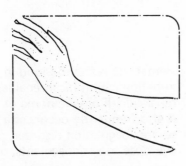

Petechiae are small red spots approximately the size of a pin head. These spots represent blood which has extravasated from intact blood vessels due to an abnormal permeability of these blood vessels. Petechiae usually occur in crops over various parts of the body, and are seen in patients with vascular disorders, in patients with thrombocytopenia and with platelet function defects. They occur in the latter two conditions because platelets are important for the maintenance of normal vascular integrity.

Purpura

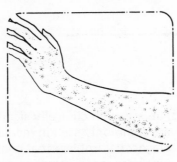

When petechiae become confluent they are known as purpura. They are larger and caused by the same abnormalities that produce petechiae.

Ecchymosis

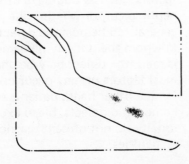

An ecchymosis or bruise is a large area of extravasated blood which usually arises from blood vessels as a result of trauma. Bruises may occur in patients who have vascular or platelet disorders.

Hematoma

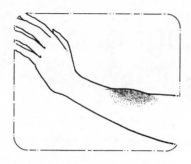

A hematoma is a large bruise which has infiltrated subcutaneous tissue or muscle and produces deformity, as well as the usual skin discolouration which is produced by a bruise. A hematoma may occur when there is a defect in the coagulation mechanism. They may be seen for instance complicating leukemia, or in hemophilia, or in pathological fibrinolysis or as a result of an overdose of oral anticoagulants.

Hemarthrosis

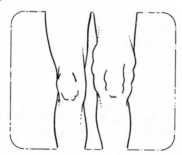

Hemarthrosis is a hemorrhage into a joint and is usually seen in patients with severe coagulation disorders, such as hemophiliacs.

Hematuria

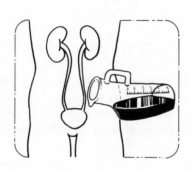

Hematuria refers to blood in urine. It occurs in patients with local renal lesions, such as renal calculi or carcinoma of the kidney, but it also frequently occurs as a result of a severe coagulation disorder, particularly overdose of anticoagulants, or hemophilia.

The Diagnostic Problem

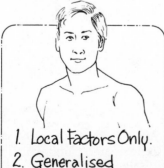

1. Local Factors Only.
2. Generalised Hemostatic Defect.
3. Hemostatic Defect unmasked by Local Factors.

Patients with clinically significant bleeding are commonly seen in medical practice. The diagnostic problem that confronts the physician is to determine whether or not the patient is bleeding as a result of local factors, such as trauma, a carcinoma, or peptic ulcer, or whether the patient has a generalized hemostatic defect. In patients in whom the underlying hemostatic defect is mild, the defect may be unmasked by local factors or may occur only after trauma. On the other hand, patients with severe hemostatic defects, bleed excessively and usually do not present diagnostic difficulties.

Approach

> 1. History.
> 2. Physical Examination.
> 3. Screening Tests.
> 4. Special Tests.

The approach to a patient with a suspected diagnosis of generalized bleeding, includes the following:

1) an adequate history,

2) careful physical examination,

3) screening tests of hemostatis and,

4) in certain circumstances, special tests of hemostasis.

History and examination will be considered in this chapter, and the Laboratory diagnosis of bleeding disorders will be considered in the next.

History

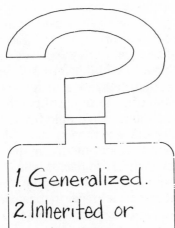

> 1. Generalized.
> 2. Inherited or Acquired.
> 3. Vascular, Platelet or Coagulation Defect.
> 4. Precise Nature & Extent of Defect.

The clinical history is probably the most important single factor in the diagnosis of a generalized bleeding disorder and in every case the bleeding symptoms should be carefully evaluated by obtaining a detailed clinical history.

Answers to the following four questions should be sought.

1) Has the patient a generalized hemostatic defect?

2) Is it inherited or acquired?

3) Is it likely to be due to a vascular or platelet abnormality, a coagulation abnormality, or a mixture of the two?

4) What is the precise nature and extent of the abnormality?

The answers to the first three questions can often be obtained by careful evaluation of the patient's bleeding manifestations, while the answer to the fourth question can only be provided by performing tests of hemostatis. Although these four questions are closely interconnected, it is useful to consider them separately.

Generalized Defect ?

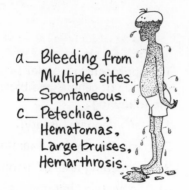

a — Bleeding from Multiple sites.
b — Spontaneous.
c — Petechiae, Hematomas, Large bruises, Hemarthrosis.

Is the patient suffering from a generalized hemostatic defect?

It is likely that the patient is suffering from a generalized hemostatic defect, if bleeding occurs from multiple sites, if it is spontaneous and if it takes the form of petechiae, hematomas, large bruises and hemarthrosis. On the other hand, it should be noted that nose bleeding, uterine bleeding and gastrointestinal bleeding are frequently caused by local factors and even when they occur in combination may not be a manifestation of a generalized bleeding abnormality.

Inherited or Acquired ?

The second question is, "Is the disorder inherited or acquired?"

Inherited

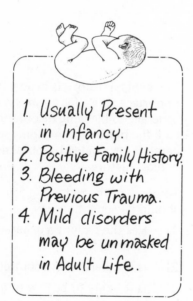

1. Usually Present in Infancy.
2. Positive Family History.
3. Bleeding with Previous Trauma.
4. Mild disorders may be unmasked in Adult Life.

Patients with inherited disorders usually present in infancy or childhood, often have a family history of bleeding and will often give a history of bleeding in response to previous operations or trauma.

The exceptions to this are patients who have inherited mild hemostatic defects and these patients may present for the first time in adult life, often with post-operative bleeding. When a patient with a mild bleeding disorder presents for the first time in adult life with either post-operative or post-traumatic bleeding, it may be difficult to decide whether the patient has a mild inherited bleeding disorder or if the disorder has recently been acquired. Differentiation between these two possibilities may sometimes be obtained by detailed enquiry of the patient's family history and enquiry into the patient's response to previous operations or episodes of trauma.

Family History (Recessive)

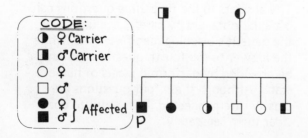

CODE:
◐ ♀ Carrier
◧ ♂ Carrier
○ ♀
□ ♂
● ♀ } Affected
■ ♂ }

This is the pattern of inheritance that is seen in an autosomal recessive trait. Neither mother or father have the disease, but are carriers, while a sibling of the propositus has the disease, & two others are carriers.

18

Family History (Dominant)

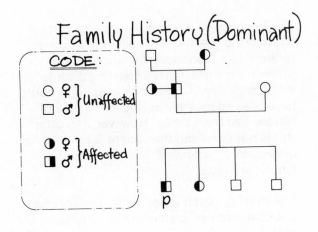

CODE:

○ ♀ } Unaffected
□ ♂ }

◐ ♀ } Affected
◧ ♂ }

This is a typical pattern of an autosomal dominant mode of inheritance, in this case the disease is transmitted by the father of the propositus, whose sister and mother also have evidence of a bleeding disorder, and one of the siblings also is affected with a bleeding disorder. A detailed family history may not only help to establish the hereditary nature of the condition, but may narrow down the number of diagnostic possibilities. In obtaining the family history every effort should be made to interview as many of the patient's relatives as possible and to obtain a detailed history from these relatives.

It should be emphasized that a positive family history of bleeding is of great value in diagnosis, but a negative history does not exclude the possibility of an inherited bleeding disorder, particularly if the family history is only obtained from the patient, or if the number of members of the family, in which a family history is available, is small.

> **Note:**
> Negative History does not exclude Hereditary Disorder.

RESPONSE TO TRAUMA

BLEEDING FROM UMBILICAL CORD

CIRCUMCISION

BRUISING

ABDOMINAL OPERATIONS

TOOTH EXTRACTIONS

TONSILLECTOMY

A careful assessment of previous response to trauma is important. This may not only strengthen the possibility that the patient is suffering from a bleeding disorder, but it may also be possible to date the onset of the disorder by careful assessment of the patient's response to previous operations or trauma. Specific enquiry should be made about bleeding from the umbilical cord at birth, bleeding after circumcision, about tooth extractions, tonsillectomy and abdominal operations. In addition, the response to the patient's previous trauma should be assessed in detail. If tonsillectomy or abdominal operations have been tolerated without excessive blood loss, it makes it unlikely that the patient is suffering from a severe or even moderately severe inherited bleeding disorder.

Acquired

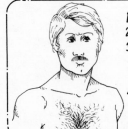

1. Generalised Bleeding
2. No Family History
3. No abnormal bleeding with previous Trauma or Operation.
4. Onset usually in Adult life.
5. Associated Disease

Most acquired hemostatic defects first present in adult life. In many cases there is an obvious underlying disorder such as liver or kidney disease, but occasionally the patient is otherwise well. The absence of bleeding with previous operative trauma and the absence of a family history strengthens the possibility that the abnormality is acquired.

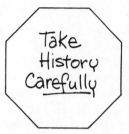

Take
History
Carefully

The importance of history taking cannot be stressed too greatly. Most patients who are referred to a laboratory for work up, do not suffer from a generalized bleeding disorder and in the majority of these, this possibility could have been adequately excluded if a careful history had been taken. However, too often this is not done and the patient is referred for unnecessary, expensive, and time-consuming laboratory tests.

Vascular, Platelet, or Coagulation Defect ?

The third question asked is, ''Is the disorder due to a vascular, platelet or coagulation defect?''

Vascular-Platelet DEFECT	Coagulation DEFECT.
1. Petechiae & Superficial Bruises.	1. Deep Spreading Hematoma.
2. Skin & Mucous Membranes.	2. Hemarthrosis.
3. Spontaneous.	3 Retroperitoneal Bleeding.
4. Bleeding immediate; prolonged, non-recurrent.	4. Bleeding prolonged & often recurrent.

The bleeding manifestations of patients with vascular disorders, thrombocyotpenia or thrombocytopathia, that is platelet function disorders, include spontaneous skin and mucous membrane bleeding, petechiae and superficial bruising. Bleeding usually starts within seconds of the injury and continues for hours, but once it stops it does not usually recur. In contrast, patients with coagulation defects develop deep-spreading hematomas, bleeding into joints, hematuria and retroperitoneal bleeding. Post-traumatic bleeding tends to be delayed, sometimes for hours after the traumatic episode and then may recur at a later time for up to 4 or 5 days.

Laboratory
Tests

Although the cause of the underlying bleeding disorder may be strongly suspected from the history and nature of bleeding manifestations, laboratory tests are required to make a precise diagnosis and these tests are the subject of the next chapter.

Self-Evaluation for Chapter 2

1. What are the characteristics of:

    petechiae,

    purpura,

    a bruise,

    a hematoma?

2. What are the features in the patient's history that make one suspect

    a)   an inherited hemostatic defect,

    b)   an acquired hemostatic defect?

3. How do the bleeding manifestations of the coagulation defect differ from those of a platelet or vascular defect?

Platelet & Vascular	Coagulation
1	1
2	2
3	3
4	4

4. What type of family history would you expect to elicit in a patient with an autosomal recessive bleeding disorder?

5. If a patient had a bleeding disorder with an autosomal dominant mode of inheritance, what percentage of his offspring would be affected with the disorder?

Chapter 3

Laboratory Diagnosis of Bleeding Disorders

Types of Tests

A. Screening Tests for Vascular & Platelet Disorders.

B. Screening Tests for Coagulation Disorders.

C. Special Tests.

Although the presence of a generalized bleeding disorder can usually be correctly suspected on the basis of history and physical examination, laboratory investigations are required to pinpoint the severity and nature of the underlying disorder. These tests can conveniently be divided into 1) screening tests for a vascular and platelet disorder, 2) screening tests for a coagulation disorder and, 3) special tests. The tests used in any individual patient are determined by the nature of the bleeding manifestations and by the clinical circumstances. It should be emphasized again that no laboratory tests or combination of laboratory tests can ever substitute for an adequate history.

Screening Tests for   *1.* Vascular *2.* Platelet Disorders

Principles

1. Evidence of Increased Vascular Fragility.
2. Evidence of Impaired Primary Hemostatic plug formation.
3. Cause of underlying disorder.

Screening Tests
1. Tourniquet Test.
2. Bleeding Time
3. Inspection of Blood Film.
4. Platelet Count.

The screening tests for vascular or platelet disorders are usually considered together because the clinical manifestations of these disorders are similar.

The approach to the patient with a suspected vascular or platelet disorder is to look for evidence of increased vascular fragility by performing a tourniquet test, remembering that increased vascular fragility is obtained in patients with vascular disorders and also in patients with thrombocytopenia and platelet function disorders, because platelets are important for the maintenance of normal vascular integrity. Secondly, to look for evidence of impaired primary hemostatic plug formation by performing a bleeding time test to look for the underlying cause of the vascular or platelet disorder.

Tourniquet Test

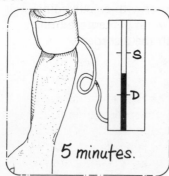

5 minutes.

The tourniquet test is performed by applying a blood pressure cuff to midway between systolic and diastolic pressure for 5 minutes, and then observing the arm distal to the cuff for evidence of petechiae. A positive tourniquet test is characteristically seen in patients with thrombocytopenia, with certain vascular disorders and with platelet function defects. However, the test is relatively non-specific.

Bleeding Time

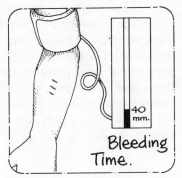

Bleeding Time.

The bleeding time is measured by determining the time required for bleeding to cease from incised small subcutaneous vessels. One method of performing this test is illustrated. This is known as the Template bleeding time test.

The blood pressure cuff is applied and inflated to 40 mm. of mercury, three standard incisions are then made on the anterior aspect of the patient's arm and the time taken for bleeding to cease is measured.

> BLEEDING TIME =
> Index of Hemostatic
> Plug formation.

The bleeding time is an index of the early stages of hemostatic plug formation.

> 1. Abnormal Vessel Constriction.
> 2. Low Platelet Count.
> 3. Abnormal Platelet Adhesion.
> 4. Abnormal Platelet release of ADP.
> 5. Abnormal Platelet Aggregation.
> 6. Abnormal Availability of Platelet Factor III.

Thus, it is prolonged in patients with abnormalities of vessel contraction, in patients with low platelet counts, abnormal adhesion of platelets to collagen, abnormal release of ADP, abnormal aggregation with ADP and abnormal platelet factor III availability.

> BLEEDING TIME
> NORMAL IN PURE
> COAGULATION DEFECT.
> WHY?

The bleeding time is usually normal in patients with coagulation disorders. This may seem surprising and perhaps difficult to explain.

> BECAUSE:

It is probable that the primary platelet plug is adequate to obtain hemostasis in the small vessels that are severed when the bleeding time is performed, or that sufficient thrombin is formed by the extrinsic pathway to stabilize the initial platelet plug and that is all that is required to achieve hemostasis when those small vessels are cut. However, if large vessels are incised, bleeding is prolonged in patients with pure coagulation defects.

> BLEEDING TIME ASSESSES:
> Vascular } Disorders.
> Platelet
>
> Normal IVY
> Bleeding Time:
> 2-6 minutes.

The bleeding time is a useful test because it gives an overall indication of the severity of hemostatic defects in patients with vascular or platelet disorders. The normal range for the Ivy bleeding time is 2 to 6 minutes.

Blood Film

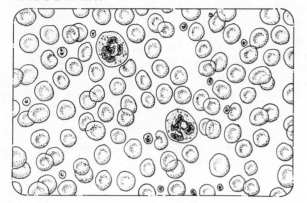

Careful inspection of the blood film may reveal the presence of an underlying cause of the thrombocytopenia, may give an indication of the platelet count and may reveal the presence of large platelets which are sometimes seen in patients with thrombocytopenia associated with rapid platelet turnover. This is a normal blood film and you can see several platelets in this field.

Platelet Count

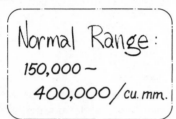

Normal Range:
150,000 –
400,000/cu.mm.

The normal range of the platelet count is 150,000 – 400,000/cu.mm. There is no absolute relationship between the platelet count and the incidence or severity of bleeding.

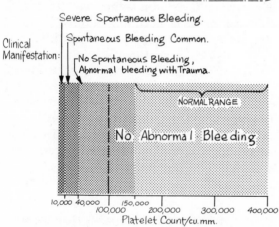

However, in general, when the platelet count is above 40,000/cu.mm. spontaneous bleeding is uncommon and serious bleeding usually occurs only after trauma or when there is a local lesion present. Bleeding is common, but not always present when the platelet count is below 40,000/cu.mm. but it is the rule, and usually severe when the platelet count is less than 10,000/cu.mm. If spontaneous bleeding does occur when the platelet count is above 40,000/cu.mm. the possibility of an associated platelet function defect or coagulation defect should be considered.

Screening Tests for Coagulation Disorders

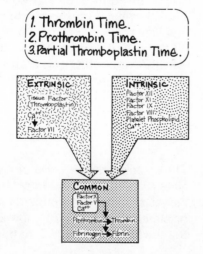

1. Thrombin Time.
2. Prothrombin Time.
3. Partial Thromboplastin Time.

The screening tests for coagulation disorders include the thrombin time, the prothrombin time and the partial thromboplastin time.

Remind yourself of the coagulation pathways. You will recall that there is an intrinsic pathway, an extrinsic pathway and a pathway common to both the intrinsic and extrinsic systems. Essentially, the screening tests for coagulation disorders are designed to detect a significant abnormality in one or more of the clotting factors and to localize this abnormality to various steps in the coagulation pathway.

Thrombin Time

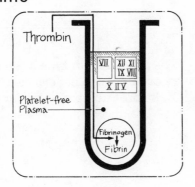

The thrombin time is performed by adding thrombin to blood or plasma. Clotting is, therefore, initiated at the fibrinogen to fibrin conversion reaction and all the other steps in the coagulation sequence are by-passed.

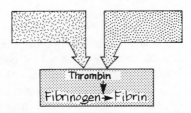

A normal thrombin time is, therefore, obtained in patients with defects of any of the coagulation factors in the intrinsic pathway, extrinsic pathway, or common pathway prior to the conversion of Fibrinogen to Fibrin.

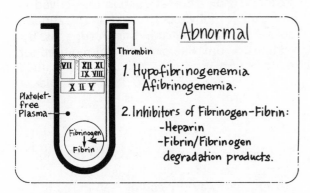

The thrombin time is abnormal in patients with low fibrinogen levels. This is otherwise known as hypofibrinogenemia or when the fibrinogen is absent from the plasma, afibrinogenemia, and in patients who have inhibitors of the fibrinogen to fibrin conversion reaction. These inhibitors include heparin and degradation products of fibrin and fibrinogen. I'll refer to the fibrinogen/fibrin degradation products again in the slide/tape show on fibrinolysis.

Prothrombin Time

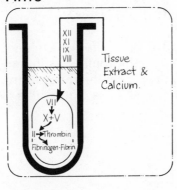

The second screening test is the prothrombin time. The prothrombin time is performed by adding tissue extract and calcium to plasma. This initiates clotting by activating factor VII which in turn activates factor X which in the presence of factor V, converts prothrombin to thrombin and the thrombin which is so produced converts fibrinogen to fibrin.

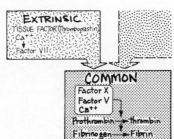

The prothrombin time, therefore, bypasses the intrinsic clotting pathway and is normal in patients with deficiencies of factors XII, XI, IX and VIII.

25

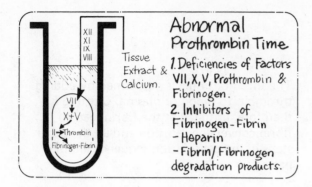

The prothrombin time is, therefore, abnormal in patients with deficiencies of factors VII, X, V, prothrombin or fibrinogen.

Partial Thromboplastin Time

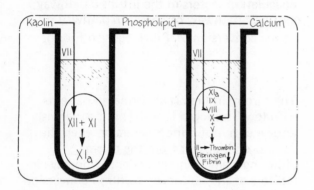

The third of the screening tests for coagulation is the partial thromboplastin time. This is performed by adding first Kaolin and then phospholipid to plasma.

Kaolin activates factors XII and XI. Phospholipid substitutes for platelets in the activation of factor VIII by factor XI, and in the activation of factor X by factors IX, VIII and V. Blood coagulation is initiated in this clotting test by adding calcium. Factor VII is not required for this reaction.

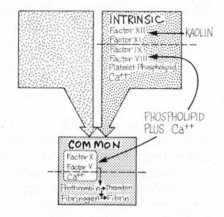

This is the pathway for the partial thromboplastin time. Essentially this is the intrinsic clotting pathway. By adding Kaolin, factors XII and XI are activated and phospholipid accelerates the reactions involved with factors VIII and factor V.

The one factor which is not affected by the partial thromboplastin time, is factor VII and the partial thromboplastin time is, therefore, normal in patients with a factor VII deficiency.

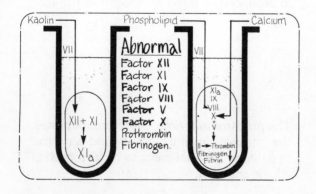

The partial thromboplastin time would be abnormal if there were deficiencies of factors XII, XI, IX, VIII, X, V, prothrombin or fibrinogen.

Test	Measures Integrity of
Thrombin Time	Fibrinogen/Fibrin Conversion
Prothrombin T.	Extrinsic Pathway
Partial Thromboplastin Time	Intrinsic Pathway

Abnormal Test	Measures Integrity of
Prothrombin Time & Partial T. Time	Multiple defects. Defect in Common Pathway.
Thrombin Time & Prothrombin Time & Partial T. Time	Fibrinogen → Fibrin alone or plus other Factor Defects.

Special Tests

1. Coagulation Factor Assays.
2. Platelet function Tests.
3. Tests for an Inhibitor.

In summary, by performing these screening tests, it is possible to localize the coagulation factor deficiency to the fibrinogen/fibrin conversion step measured by the thrombin time, to the extrinsic pathway measured by the prothrombin time, and the intrinsic pathway measured by the partial thromboplastin time.

A combined abnormality of the prothrombin and partial thromboplastin time would indicate either multiple defects involving both pathways or a defect in the common pathway.

An abnormality of all three screening tests would indicate an abnormality in the fibrinogen to fibrin reaction either alone or in combination with other defects.

Special tests include coagulation factor assays to identify precisely the nature of the coagulation defect, platelet function tests, and tests for a circulating inhibitor.

Self Evaluation for Chapter 3

1. What are the disorders associated with a prolonged bleeding time?

2. Why is the bleeding time normal in hemophilia?

3. When is the thrombin time abnormally long?

4. Is the thrombin time normal or abnormally long in hemophilia?

5. What are the coagulation factors that are measured by the prothrombin time?

6. What are the coagulation factors that are measured by the partial thromboplastin time?

7. What are the coagulation disorders that will produce a long prothrombin time and a long partial thromboplastin time?

Chapter 4

Vascular Disorders

Causes of Abnormal Bleeding

| VASCULAR DISORDERS |
| Thrombocytopenia |
| Platelet·Function Defects |
| Coagulation Defects |
| Fibrinolysis |

The diagnosis of a vascular defect is usually made after thrombocytopenia and a qualitative platelet defect have been excluded.

Vascular Disorders

CHARACTERISTICS:
- Easy Bruising.
- Spontaneous Bleeding.

The vascular disorders are a heterogeneous group of conditions which are characterized by easy bruising and spontaneous bleeding from the small vessels.

Defects in Blood Vessels

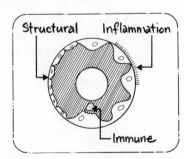

Structural   Inflammation

Immune

The underlying abnormality is thought to be either in the vessels themselves eg: structurally weak vessels, or vessels damaged by inflammation or immune processes, or to abnormality in the perivascular connective tissue. Vascular defects are the commonest cause of bleeding disorders seen in clinical practice.

Manifestations

CLINICAL:
1. Bleeding often not severe.
2. Mainly bleeding into skin.
3. Bleeding occurs immediately after Trauma.

Most cases of bleeding due to a vascular defect alone are not severe. Frequently the bleeding is mainly or wholly in the skin, causing petechiae or ecchymoses or both. In some disorders there is also bleeding from mucous membranes. Excess bleeding from wounds tends to occur at once, usually persists for less than 48 hours, and rarely recurs.

In some of these conditions the standard screening tests used in the investigation of patients with a bleeding disorder show little or no abnormality. The bleeding time is rarely prolonged but the tourniquet test may be positive.

Inherited or Acquired

The vascular defects may be inherited or acquired.

Hereditary:

Hemorrhagic Telangiectasia

1. Autosomal Dominant.
2. Abnormal dilated blood Vessels.
3. Epistaxis.
4. Iron Deficiency.

The most common hemorrhagic disorder which is clearly caused by an inherited vascular abnormality is hereditary hemorrhagic telangiectasia.

It is an uncommon disorder transmitted as an autosomal dominant trait and it, therefore, affects both sexes equally. The basic lesion is the presence in the skin and mucous membranes of telangiectases due to multiple dilatations of capillaries and arterioles. The telangiectases are lined by a thin layer of endothelial cells. Because of their thinness, they bleed easily, and because they contract poorly the bleeding is often prolonged. Bleeding often does not occur until early adult life and epistaxis is the commonest symptom and usually the presenting manifestation. Anemia not uncommonly occurs due to chronic blood loss and iron deficiency. The tourniquet test and bleeding time are usually normal.

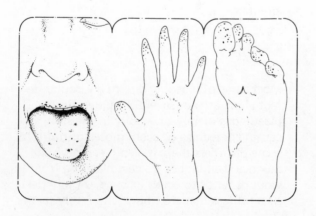

The commonest sites of lesions are the skin and mucous membranes of nose and mouth, however, they may also occur at other sites. Lesions in the skin are mainly seen on the face and on the tips of fingers and on the feet. In the mouth they occur on the lips, tongue, cheeks and palate. The lesions blanch on pressure and tend to become more numerous and larger with advancing age.

Acquired Vascular Defects

> 1. Simple Easy Bruising.
> 2. Senile Purpura.
> 3. Infections & Drugs.
> 4. Henoch Schonlein Syndrome.
> 5. Scurvy.
> 6. Corticosteroids.

The acquired vascular defects to be considered here are: simple easy bruising, senile purpura, infections and drugs, Henoch Schonlein Syndrome, scurvy and corticosteroid administration.

Simple Bruising

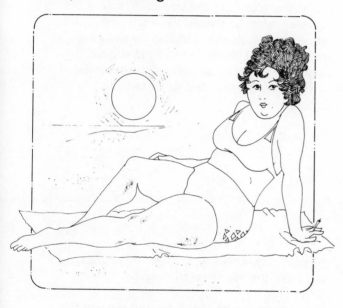

Simple easy bruising is a common benign disorder which occurs predominantly in otherwise healthy women, especially those of childbearing age. The onset is often during adolescence or early adult life.

The disorder is relatively common and is characterized by the recurrence of circumscribed bruises, either on minor trauma or without obvious cause. These are most often seen on the legs and trunk. The bruises are occasionally preceded by pain due to rupture of small blood vessels.

The cause of the disorder is unknown, but is likely due to increased fragility of skin vessels. It is only of importance because of its cosmetic significance and because it may give rise to suspicions of a serious blood disorder. It is probably the commonest cause of referral of patients for diagnosis and assessment of unexplained skin bruising.

> DIAGNOSIS
> by exclusion:
>
> NORMAL:
> Bleeding Time & Tourniquet Tests.
> Ask re.:
> Aspirin Ingestion.

Diagnosis is made on clinical features and by excluding other causes of purpura. There are no abnormalities of any of the special tests related to bleeding disorders, that is, the bleeding time and tourniquet test are usually normal. A history of aspirin ingestion should be sought, as this may give a similar bruising condition or aggravate bruising in patients with simple easy bruising. The disorder does not cause excessive bleeding at operation, and there is sometimes a family history.

Senile Purpura

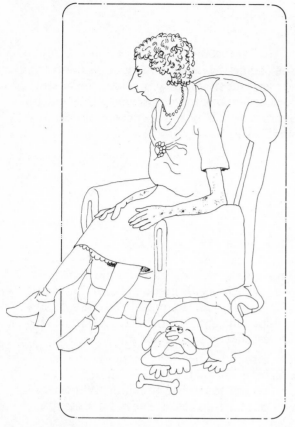

Senile purpura is a form of purpura which occurs commonly in elderly subjects. The purpura occurs mainly in the extensor aspect of the forearms and hands. The lesion does not occur on other parts of the body although they are occasionally seen on the face in relationship to spectacle frames.

The purpuric areas are large, irregular, dark purple and have a clear-cut margin. The skin in the affected parts is inelastic, smooth and thin. Histological section of the skin in the affected areas shows marked atrophy of collagen, this results in the skin being freely movable over the deeper tissues. The purpuric lesions are thus easily induced by shearing strain to the skin which tears the vessels passing to the skin because of the excessive mobility of the skin and subcutaneous tissues.

Infections & Drugs

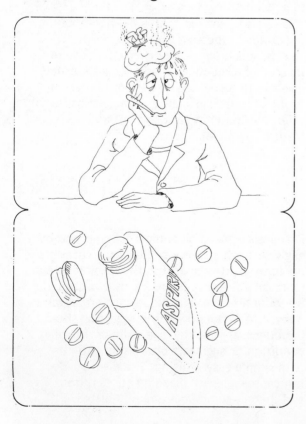

Purpura may occur with many infections, and after the ingestion of drugs.

The purpura caused by infection is generally considered to be due to microthrombi and toxic damage of the vascular endothelium. However, it is being increasingly recognized that disseminated intravascular thrombosis and consumption coagulopathy may be present and contribute to the bleeding tendency. Occasionally purpura is the first manifestation of an occult infection particularly in children. A number of drugs have been reported to cause purpura, occasionally with mucous membrane bleeding. The purpura usually clears within a few days of stopping the drug and commonly recurs if the drug is readministered. Some of the drugs which cause vascular purpura also cause thrombocytopenic purpura.

Henoch Schonlein Syndrome

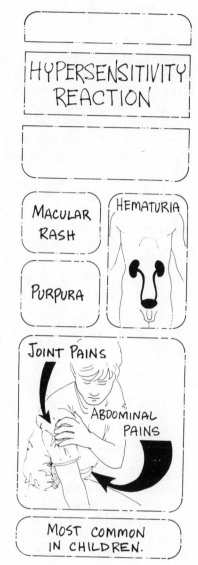

The Henoch Schonlein Syndrome is thought to be a hypersensitivity reaction with a fundamental disturbance of widespread acute inflammation of the capillaries and small arterioles. This results in increased vascular permeability and thus in exudation and hemorrhage into the tissues.

Clinically it presents as an acute condition characterized by a macular rash, purpura, joint pains, gastrointestinal pain, and hematuria. The condition occurs most commonly in children, but may occur in adults. It is usually self-limiting, but may recur for a period of up to 2 to 3 months. The onset may follow an upper respiratory tract infection, often with a Group A, beta hemolytic streptococcus. It may occur following the ingestion of certain drugs, but most often no cause is found.

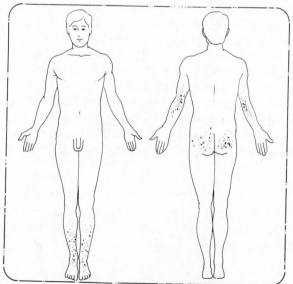

The purpuric rash occurs most commonly on the buttocks, on the backs of the elbows and extensor surfaces of the arms, on the extensor surface of the lower leg, the ankle and the foot. It is usually bilateral. It may occur in crops which progressively fade over weeks, but occasionally it is frankly hemorrhagic.

Scurvy

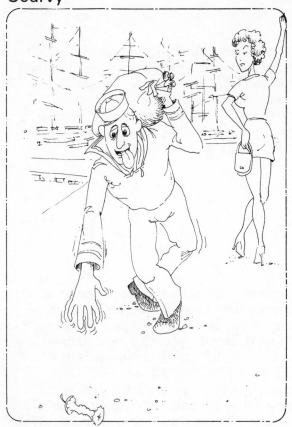

Hemorrhage is a common feature of scurvy, which is caused by Vitamin C deficiency.

It is primarily due to an increased vascular fragility which results from defective formation of the intracellular substance of the vascular wall. Vitamin C is necessary for normal collagen formation.

The skin is the commonest site of hemorrhage, which occurs as both petechiae and ecchymoses of various sizes. Hemorrhage is particularly common in the legs and at sites of trauma. Petechiae are commonly perifollicular, that is, surrounding hair follicles. The bleeding time is often prolonged and the tourniquet test is usually positive.

Cushing's Disease

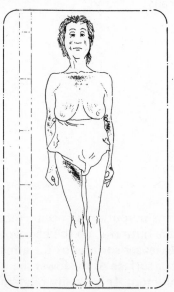

Bruising is a common feature of Cushing's Disease, that is, an over-secretion of corticosteroid hormones and is also a common feature of patients who were treated with large doses of corticosteroids for prolonged periods of time.

Patients may show bruising or multiple petechial hemorrhages and purpuric spots over the body. The disorder appears to be due to a vascular defect due possibly to the fact that patients with Cushing's Disease, or those treated with high doses of steroids for long periods of time, lose subcutaneous tissue which normally supports vessels coursing between muscles and skin. These vessels therefore readily bleed, even with mild trauma.

Self Evaluation for Chapter 4

1. What are the clinical manifestations of vascular disorders?

    — — — — — — — — — — — — — — — — —

    — — — — — — — — — — — — — — — —

    — — — — — — — — — — — — — —

2. List the common vascular disorders.

    — — — — — — — — — — — — — — —

    — — — — — — — — — — — — — — — —

    — — — — — — — — — — — — — — —

    — — — — — — — — — — — — — —

    — — — — — — — — — — — — — —

    — — — — — — — — — — — — — —

Chapter 5

Platelet Disorders

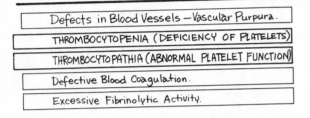

Defects in Blood Vessels – Vascular Purpura.
THROMBOCYTOPENIA (DEFICIENCY OF PLATELETS)
THROMBOCYTOPATHIA (ABNORMAL PLATELET FUNCTION)
Defective Blood Coagulation.
Excessive Fibrinolytic Activity.

Platelet function may be impaired because of a fall in the number of circulating platelets, known as Thrombocytopenia or because of a platelet function abnormality.

Vascular Defects.
THROMBOCYTOPENIA.
Platelet Function Defects.
Coagulation Defects.
Fibrinolysis.

Before going into the pathogenesis of thrombocytopenia, the normal physiology of platelet production and destruction will be briefly reviewed.

Megakaryocyte Development

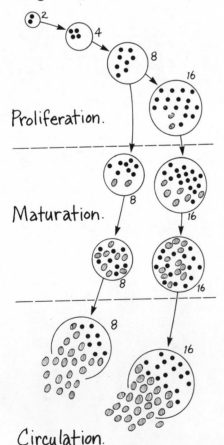

This diagram shows megakaryocyte development and platelet formation. Megakaryocytes are multinucleated precursors of platelets which are found in the bone marrow. They arise from mononuclear precursors which characteristically undergo nuclear replication without cytoplasmic replication. Therefore, the cells are multinucleate. As a result, the amount of DNA material in the cell increases, and while doing so, the size of the cell increases. Three stages in megakaryocyte development are recognized. The first is nuclear proliferation, and during this stage, the nuclei, shown as black dots, undergo replication. At the eighth nuclear stage, cytoplasmic maturation begins and this cytoplasmic maturation is characterized by the appearance of granules in the cytoplasm. These granules represent platelet precursors. During cytoplasmic maturation membranes form which demarcate the cytoplasm into platelet sub-units and after maturation is completed, the mass of preformed platelets is released from the megakaryocytes into the blood stream. The number of platelets produced by megakaryocytes is proportional to the amount of cytoplasm. In the normal marrow about 25% of the megakaryocytes are immature, containing no apparent granules and the other 75% show varying degrees of maturity, that is varying degrees of granulation.

Thrombopoietin

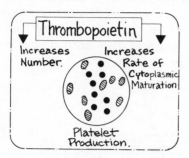

Platelet production is under the control of a humoral agent which is known as thrombopoietin. The site of synthesis of thrombopoietin is unknown, but there is good evidence that thrombopoietin synthesis is stimulated by thrombocytopenic states and that the thrombopoietin acts both to increase the number of megakaryocytes formed from precursor cells and to increase the rate of cytoplasmic maturation and platelet release.

Platelet Kinetics

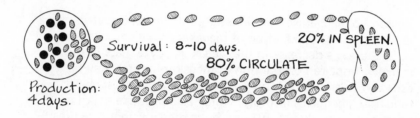

After release from the megakaryocytes, platelets circulate as cytoplasmic discs in a concentration of approximately 250,000 platelets per cu. mm. of blood. The volume of platelets diminishes as they mature in the circulation. Thus, young platelets are larger than old platelets. About 80% of the platelets circulate within the blood stream and the remainder are pooled in the spleen. The platelet life span is approximately 10 days.

Recent evidence suggests that young platelets may spend up to 24 - 36 hours in the spleen after being discharged from the bone marrow. Splenic enlargement, otherwise known as splenomegaly is associated with a marked increase in splenic pooling, so that as much as 80% — 90% of the body platelets may be pooled in the spleen, in someone with splenic enlargement. A marked increase in platelet requirements, (for example, due to accelerated destruction of platelets) can provoke the release of platelets prematurely from the marrow and these platelets are larger than normal.

Causes of Thrombocytopenia

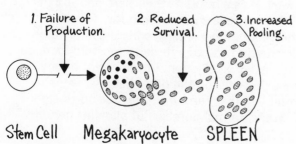

It follows from what has been said, that thrombocytopenia may occur as a result of (1) decreased platelet production, as a result of (2) an increased rate of platelet destruction, or (3) as a result of increased splenic platelet pooling, which is associated with splenomegaly.

1. Failure of Production

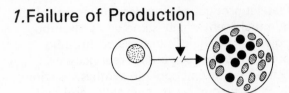

Decreased platelet production may result from a reduced number of megakaryocytes in the marrow, or from ineffective platelet production from normal numbers of mega-karyocytes.

Decreased Production.

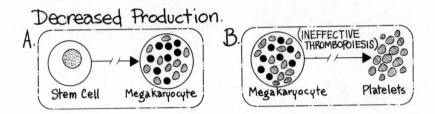

A. Stem Cell → Megakaryocyte

B. (INEFFECTIVE THROMBOPOIESIS) Megakaryocyte → Platelets

These two mechanisms are illustrated. In thrombocyotpenia due to impaired production of megakaryocytes from stem cells, there is a decrease in the megakaryocyte mass in the marrow. Impaired production of megakaryocytes may be caused by agents which produce marrow damage, such as radiation, chemicals or drugs, which also produce aplastic anemia, may be due to intrinsic bone marrow abnormalities such as leukemia, or may be caused by replacement of bone marrow with carcinoma cells or with plasma cells in a condition known as multiple myeloma. Ineffective platelet production from megakaryocytes, otherwise known as ineffective thrombopoiesis is seen in patients with megaloblastic anemias in whom there is a normal megakaryocyte mass, but a marked decrease in platelet production per megakaryocyte unit.

2. Increased Destruction

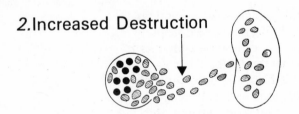

The second cause of thrombocytopenia is increased rate of destruction. There are two mechanisms of increased rate of destruction in circulating blood.

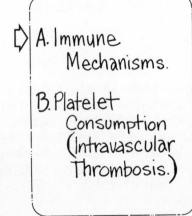

A. Immune Mechanisms.

B. Platelet Consumption (Intravascular Thrombosis.)

The first is an immune mechanism due to damage of platelets by platelet antibodies, and the second is due to consumption of platelets as a result of their participation in diffuse intravascular thrombosis. Acute thrombocytopenia due to increased platelet destruction causes a three to fourfold increase in platelet production. Chronic thrombocy-topenic states on the other hand, are able to stimulate the marrow to produce up to eight-fold the normal numbers of platelets per day.

Immune Thrombocytopenia

> A. Chronic.
> B. Acute.
> C. Drug Induced.

Three forms of immune thrombocytopenia are recognized clinically. The first is chronic immune thrombocytopenia the second is acute thrombocytopenia, and the third is drug induced immune thrombocytopenia.

Chronic Immune Thrombocytopenia

> A. IDIOPATHIC
> B. SECONDARY:
>   -Disseminated Lupus Erythematosus
>   -Hodgkin's Disease.
>   -Chronic Lymphocytic Leukemia.

Chronic immune thrombocytopenia is usually idiopathic, that is, it is usually unaccompanied by other disease, but it is also seen in association with diseases such as disseminated lupus erythematosus, Hodgkin's Disease, and chronic lymphocytic leukemia.

③ ♀ : ① ♂

Chronic immune thrombocytopenia most commonly affects young adults and is about three times more common in females than in males.

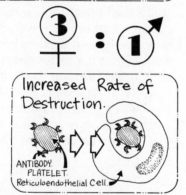

Increased Rate of Destruction.

ANTIBODY.
PLATELET.
Reticuloendothelial Cell.

In this disorder the platelets are sensitized by platelet antibodies. These antibodies are auto-antibodies and they coat the patient's platelets and sensitize them, so that they are destroyed in the reticuloendothelial tissues.

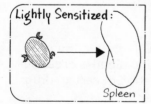

Lightly Sensitized:
Spleen

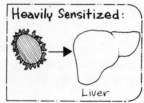

Heavily Sensitized:
Liver

Lightly sensitized platelets are mainly destroyed in the spleen while the very heavily sensitized platelets are destroyed in the liver and in other reticuloendothelial tissues throughout the body.

Treatment

1. Reduce Circulating Antibody

2. Reduce Rate of Destruction of Sensitized Platelets.

| Immuno-supressive Therapy. | STEROIDS |
| Splenectomy | |

The treatment of chronic immune thrombocytopenia is aimed at
1) reducing the level of circulating antibody and
2) reducing the rate of destruction of the sensitized platelets by the reticuloendothelial system.

Immunosuppressive therapy by drugs such as Axothioprine or Cyclophosphamide are thought to act by decreasing the titer of circulating autoantibody, while splenectomy, that is, removal of the spleen, relieves thrombocytopenia in a large percentage of these patients because it removes the principal site of destuction of sensitized platelets. Corticosteroids act at both of these levels.

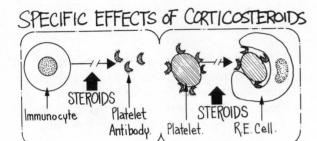

SPECIFIC EFFECTS OF CORTICOSTEROIDS

Corticosteroids act by decreasing the production of autoantibodies and also by decreasing the speed of removal or destruction of sensitized platelets by the spleen. It is likely that the latter mechanism is the more important.

Acute Immune Thrombocytopenia

1. Children.

2. 75% Post-infective.

3. ? Immune ?

The second of the immune thrombocytopenias is acute thrombocytopenia. Acute thrombocytopenia often occurs in children and is usually self-limiting. The mechanism of thrombocytopenia in the majority of patients with acute thrombocytopenia is less well understood than the chronic immune thrombocytopenic states. However, in about 75% of cases there is a preceding infection and it may well be that the thrombocytopenia represents an immune reaction to the infection. Alternatively, it is possible that platelets are destroyed as a result of interaction with the antigen/antibody complex that forms about 7-10 days after any acute viral or bacterial infection.

Drug Induced Immune Thrombocytopenia

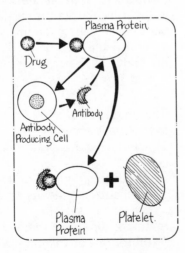

An immune reaction with destruction of platelets in the peripheral blood is occasionally seen after the ingestion of certain drugs.

The pathogenesis of drug-induced immune thrombocytopenia has recently been clarified and the mechanism is as shown here. It is likely that in most cases the drug combines with a plasma protein, to form an antigen which results in antibody formation. When the drug is readministered the antibody combines with the antigen to form an immune complex which is absorbed onto the platelet surface.

Platelet Lysis:

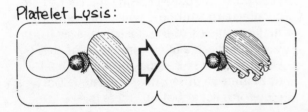

Contact of the immune complex with platelets results in platelet destruction in the circulation.

Increased Destruction

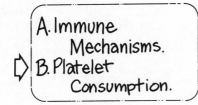

The second cause of increased rate of platelet destruction is consumption of platelets due to their participation in diffuse intravascular thrombosis.

Consumption of Platelets

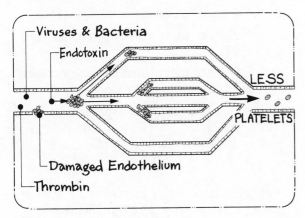

This shows some of the triggers which may produce thrombocytopenia as a result of disseminated intravascular thrombosis. These include damaged endothelium to which the platelets adhere, thrombin, viruses & bacteria, and endotoxin, all of which produce platelet aggregation. After aggregation the platelets become sequestered in arterioles and capillaries and so their level in the circulation falls.

Thrombotic Thrombocytopenic Purpura

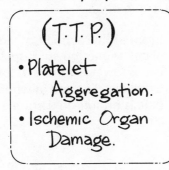

One cause of disseminated intravascular platelet aggregation is a disorder known as thrombotic thrombocytopenic purpura (T.T.P.) This is characterized by purpura due to platelet clumping in microaggregates and ischemic organ damage eg: in the kidney and brain, due to thrombosis of the microcirculation.

3. Increased Splenic Pooling

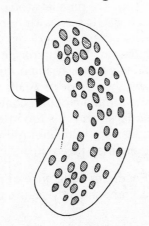

The third cause of thrombocytopenia is increased splenic pooling. There is an increase in the proportion of platelets pooled in the spleen in patients with splenic enlargement from any cause. This may result in the decreased concentration of platelets in the general circulation, if the bone marrow is not able to compensate for the increased pool size. In many of the conditions associated with increased splenic pooling there is also some reduction in platelet survival and also some impairment of platelet production, both of which contribute to the thrombocytopenia.

| Vascular Defects. |
| Thrombocytopenia. |
| **THROMBOCYTOPATHIA.** |
| Coagulation Defects. |
| Fibrinolysis. |

Disorders of platelet function are known as thrombocytopathia. As we have seen, four types of disorders of platelet function are recognized.

Hemostatic Plug Formation

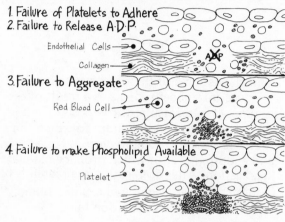

1. Failure of Platelets to Adhere
2. Failure to Release A.D.P.

    Endothelial Cells ⟶

    Collagen ⟶

3. Failure to Aggregate

    Red Blood Cell ⟶

4. Failure to make Phospholipid Available

    Platelet ⟶

1) Failure of platelets to adhere to the collagen of the damaged vessel wall.

2) Failure of platelets to release ADP.

3) Failure of platelets to aggregate with ADP.

4) Failure to make platelet phospholipid available for coagulation.

In many cases the defects may co-exist although isolated platelet function defects have been described.

> ### Platelet Function Disorders:
> Primary ⟨ Inherited / Acquired
> Secondary

Platelet disorders may be primary — that is due to a dysfunction of the platelets without evidence of associated disease, or may be secondary to a recognizable clinical disorder. The primary disorders may be inherited or acquired.

> ### Clinical Suspicions:
> • Abnormal bleeding.
> • Prolonged bleeding time.
> • Normal Platelet Count.

From a clinical point of view, disorders of platelet function are suspected in patients who show abnormal skin or mucous membrane bleeding and in whom the bleeding time is prolonged despite a normal platelet count.

Failure of Platelets to Adhere

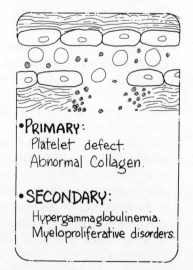

• **PRIMARY:**
Platelet defect.
Abnormal Collagen.

• **SECONDARY:**
Hypergammaglobulinemia.
Myeloproliferative disorders.

Failure of platelets to adhere to subendothelial collagen is seen with hypergammaglobulinemia when there are very high levels of gamma globulin. The gamma globulin coats the platelets interfering both with their adherence and the release of ADP. It is also possible that the gamma globulin coats the subendothelial collagen and this too interferes with platelet adhesion. In myeloproliferative disorders there may be an intrinsic platelet defect.

Failure of adherence of platelets is usually accompanied by failure of ADP release.

Failure to Release A.D.P.

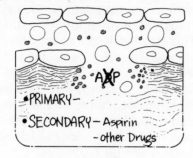

Failure to release ADP has been described as an isolated inherited disorder; or secondary to the administration of certain drugs, notably aspirin.

There is now evidence that the release reaction, that is the reaction responsible for the release of ADP from platelets, is closely linked to prostaglandin synthesis in platelets.

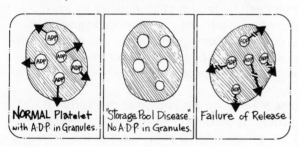

When a release reaction inducing agent such as collagen is added to platelets it activates an enzyme system which in turn results in the production of arachadonic acid from phospholipid. The arachadonic acid in turn is converted into unstable endoperoxide intermediates which are precursors of prostaglandins. Some of the endoperoxides initiate the release reaction.

Primary Platelet Release Defects

There are two types of inherited release defects. One is associated with reduced levels of ADP in platelet granules and is known as "storage pool disease". The other is associated with a failure of the release mechanism.

Aspirin Defect

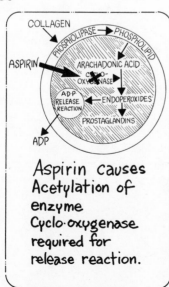

Aspirin causes Acetylation of enzyme Cyclo·oxygenase required for release reaction.

The effect of aspirin on platelets is of considerable interest because of its therapeutic implication. Aspirin works by inhibiting the release mechanism. It has been shown that although aspirin is cleared from the circulation very quickly, that is within 30 minutes of ingestion, the platelet function defect produced by aspirin lasts for up to 4 - 7 days. This is caused by the acetylation by aspirin of an enzyme cyclo-oxygenase which is present in platelets and which catalyzes the synthesis of endoperoxides and thromboxane A_2 from arrachidonic acid. The aspirin defect is characterized by inhibition of ADP release with aggregating agents such as adrenalin and collagen.

Failure to Aggregate

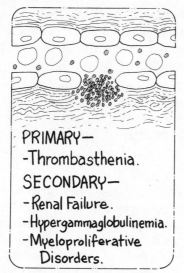

PRIMARY—
-Thrombasthenia.
SECONDARY—
-Renal Failure.
-Hypergammaglobulinemia.
-Myeloproliferative
  Disorders.

Failure of platelets to aggregate with ADP is seen in one well-defined though rare primary inherited disorder known as thrombasthenia. This may result in a severe bleeding abnormality with bruising, petechiae and purpura. Platelet aggregation is defective in renal failure. The disorder is reversible by dialysis and is, therefore, due to retained metabolites, and in particular a substance known as guanidinosuccinic acid which interferes with aggregation by ADP.

Failure of aggregation is also seen in hypergammaglobulinemia due to coating of the platelets, and in the myeloproliferative disorders probably due to an intrinsic defect of the platelets.

Failure to make Phospholipid Available

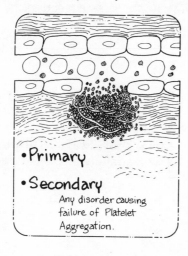

•Primary

•Secondary
  Any disorder causing
  failure of Platelet
  Aggregation.

Platelet phospholipid is normally made available when platelets aggregate. Therefore, there will be failure of availability in any disorder interfering with platelet aggregation. A qualitative defect of platelet phospholipid has been described in a number of families with bleeding disorders.

The abnormality is known as the Bernard-Soulier Syndrome. These patients usually have abnormally large platelets in the circulation.

Self Evaluation for Chapter 5

1. What are the possible mechanisms of thrombocytopenia?

    _____

    _____

    _____

2. What are the mechanisms of decreased platelet survival?

    _____

    _____

3. What is the mechanism of chronic idiopathic thrombo-
    cytopenic purpura?

    _____

    _____

    _____

4. What is the mechanism(s) of acute idiopathic thrombo-
    cytopenic purpura?

    _____

    _____

    _____

5. Name the disorders of platelet function that are
    recognized clinically.

    _____

    _____

    _____

    _____

Chapter 6

Coagulation Disorders:
General Principles

Vascular Defects.

Thrombocytopenia.

Thrombocytopathia.

COAGULATION DEFECTS.

Excessive Fibrinolysis.

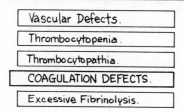

Abnormal bleeding may be caused by deficiencies of coagulation factors.

Mechanisms of Production:
Coagulation Factor Defects

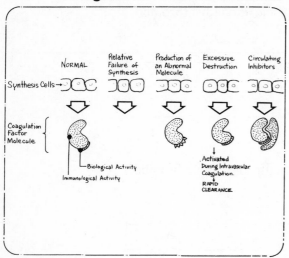

These may be produced in several ways. Firstly, there could be reduced synthesis of the coagulation factor molecule. Secondly, the coagulation factor defect could be caused by synthesis of a qualitatively abnormal molecule. Thirdly, it could be caused by loss or excessive peripheral destruction of the coagulation factors and fourthly, by inactivation of the coagulation factor by circulating antibodies.

Sites of Synthesis

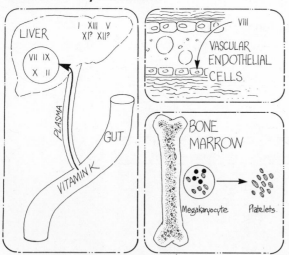

Coagulation factors VII, IX, X and prothrombin(II), fibrinogen, factors XIII, V and probably also factors XI and XII are synthesized in the liver. The hepatic synthesis of factors VII, IX, X and prothrombin is vitamin K dependent. Platelets are produced by megakaryocytes in the bone marrow. There is evidence that factor VIII antigen is synthesized in endothelial cells and that this molecule subsequently acquires coagulant activity by some unknown process.

Inherited Deficiencies

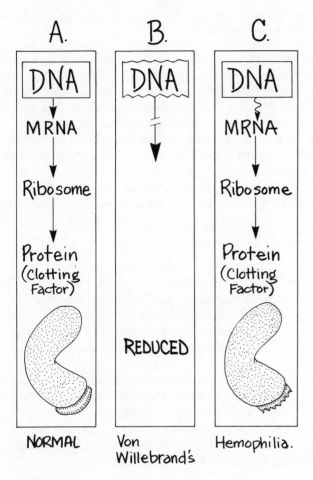

It was originally thought that the inherited deficiencies of coagulation factors were always caused by a failure of synthesis.

Evidence is now accumulating which indicates that many of these disorders are due to synthesis of abnormal molecules, and not to reduced synthesis of normal molecules.

The possibilities are represented in this diagram. The normal situation is shown in column A. Column B indicates our original concept of synthetic deficiencies, in which an inherited chromosomal abnormality (D.N.A.) leads to failure of protein synthesis.

However, as mentioned above, there is now increasing evidence that the majority of patients with hereditary coagulation factor deficiencies synthesize biologically inactive coagulation factors, which however, retain immunological reactivity as represented in Column C.

The exception is von Willebrand's disease in which there appears to be reduced synthesis of factor VIII.

Acquired Deficiencies

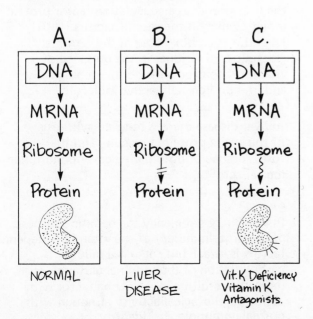

In considering acquired coagulation defects, there is evidence that patients treated with vitamin K antagonists produce biologically inactive coagulation factors which retain their immunological identity, but that the coagulation disorder encountered in liver disease is due to diminished or absent synthesis of the complete molecule.

Vitamin K Deficiency

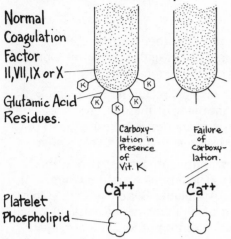

Normal Coagulation Factor II, VII, IX or X

Glutamic Acid Residues.

Carboxylation in Presence of Vit. K

Ca++

Failure of Carboxylation.

Ca++

Platelet Phospholipid

The abnormality in coagulation found in vitamin K deficiency has recently been clarified.

Synthesis of factors II, VII, IX and X is abnormal in vitamin K deficiency and following the use of vitamin K antagonists, drugs which are used therapeutically as oral anticoagulants. The factor II, VII, IX and X molecules produced are abnormal in that there is failure of carboxylation of terminal glutamic acid residues on the end of the protein molecule. This results in normal levels of immunologically detectable clotting protein, but biologically inactive protein. The biological inactivity is caused by failure of the molecule to bind calcium, and therefore, to form complexes with phospholipid.

Summary

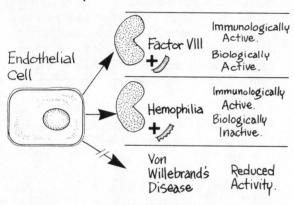

Endothelial Cell

Factor VIII + — Immunologically Active. Biologically Active.

Hemophilia + — Immunologically Active. Biologically Inactive.

Von Willebrand's Disease — Reduced Activity.

To summarize then: firstly, the synthesis of the immunologically detectable factor VIII molecule normally occurs in endothelial cells. This molecule subsequently acquires coagulant activity (becomes biologically active.)

In hemophilia an immunologically normal protein is produced by endothelial cells, but this does not acquire coagulant activity.

In von Willebrand's disease there is reduced synthesis of the entire molecule.

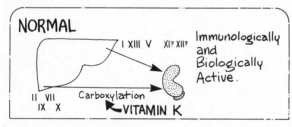

NORMAL — I XIII V XI? XII? II VII IX X — Carboxylation ←VITAMIN K — Immunologically and Biologically Active.

Secondly, the synthesis of factors I, XIII, V, II, VII, IX, and X and probably XI and XII occurs in the liver. Under normal conditions the liver produces a coagulation factor protein moiety which in the case of factors II, VII, IX and X is carboxylated at the terminal glutamic acid residues in the presence of vitamin K to produce a normal biologically and immunologically active molecule.

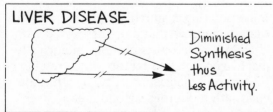

LIVER DISEASE — Diminished Synthesis thus Less Activity.

In liver disease there is reduced synthesis of the entire protein molecule, and therefore, absence of both biological and immunological activity.

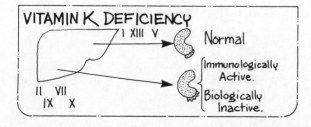

VITAMIN K DEFICIENCY — I XIII V — Normal — II VII IX X — Immunologically Active. Biologically Inactive.

In vitamin K deficiency the hepatic synthesis of the protein moiety of the Vitamin K dependent factors is intact, but there is a failure of carboxylation of the terminal glutamic acid molecule resulting in a clotting factor with abnormal biological activity although with normal immunological identity.

48

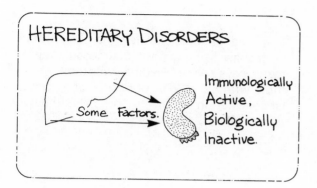

HEREDITARY DISORDERS

Some Factors. → Immunologically Active, Biologically Inactive.

The inherited disorders of the coagulation factors that are produced in the liver have not been as well characterized as hemophilia, but current evidence indicates that in some of these disorders there may be synthesis of a biologically inactive molecule which retains immunological identity.

Hereditary Deficiencies

DEFECT	MODE OF INHERITANCE	INCIDENCE
XII	Autosomal Recessive	V. Rare
XI	Autosomal Recessive	Rare
IX Christmas D.	Sex linked Recessive	Uncommon
VIII Hemophilia	Sex linked Recessive	Uncommon
VIII Von Willebrands D.	Autosomal Dominant	Uncommon
VII	Autosomal Recessive	Very Rare
X		
V		
II (Prothrombin)	AUTOSOMAL RECESSIVE	VERY RARE
I (Fibrinogen)		
XIII		

Hereditary deficiencies of each of the ten clotting factors have been described. All of these inherited coagulation disorders are uncommon, and all except Hemophilia, Christmas Disease and von Willebrand's Disease are rare. Hemophilia is about five times more common than Christmas Disease. Von Willebrand's Disease is now being recognized more frequently. Hemophilia is a factor VIII deficiency, and Christmas Disease is caused by factor IX deficiency. Both are transmitted as sex-linked recessive traits and von Willebrand's Disease, which is a factor VIII deficiency associated with a platelet abnormality, is transmitted as an autosomal dominant trait. All of the other inherited coagulation disorders are believed to be transmitted as autosomal recessives.

Correlation of Symptoms with Severity of Deficiency

DEFECT	LABORATORY DEFECT	CLINICAL DEFECT
XII	Abnormal PTT	NONE
XI	Abnormal PTT	DISPROP. MILD
IX Christmas D.	Abnormal PTT	PROPORTIONATELY SEVERE
VIII Hemophilia		
VIII Von Willebrands D.		
VII	Abnormal PT	DISPROPORTIONATELY MODERATE
X	Abnormal PTT & PT	PROPORTIONATELY SEVERE
V		
II (Prothrombin)		
I (Fibrinogen)	Abnormal P.T.T. P.T. & T.C.T.	PROP. SEVERE
XIII	Normal P.T.T. P.T. & T.C.T.	DISPROP. SEVERE

In general, there is good correlation between the severity of a patient's symptoms and the severity of the coagulation deficiency. However, there are some exceptions to this general rule. Factor XII deficiency produces a marked laboratory defect, but no clinical bleeding. Factor XI deficiency produces a marked laboratory defect, but clinical symptoms are disproportionately mild. In factor VII deficiency the clinical effects are also disproportionately less than the laboratory defects, although the discrepancy between clinical and laboratory effects is less marked than in the previous two. Finally, factor XIII deficiency produces clinical bleeding, but all of the screening tests for coagulation disorders are normal. This deficiency is diagnosed by demonstrating abnormal solubility of the fibrin clot in solvents such as urea.

Clinical Severity	Level of Clotting Factor
Severe	<1%
Moderate	1-5%
Mild	5-25%

In general patients with less than 1% of the normal level of any particular coagulation factor have severe bleeding symptoms while those with 5% to 20% of normal of a particular coagulation factor only have a mild defect seen clinically.

Catabolism of Coagulation Factors

FACTOR	½ LIFE (HOURS)
VII	4-5
V VIII	15
IX	25
X XI XII	40
II Prothrombin	60
I Fibrinogen; XIII	90
Platelets	100-120

The turnover and half-life disappearance of coagulation factors has been evaluated either by using isotopic methods or by plasma transfusion in patients with isolated deficiencies of coagulation factors. Similarly, platelet turnover has been measured by infusing labelled platelets into normal recipients.

The approximate turnover rates of coagulation factors and platelets is summarized in this Table. Factor VII has a very short half-life disappearance, being approximately 4 - 5 hours, while fibrinogen, factor XIII and platelets have a half-life disappearance of four to five days.

Blood Storage & its effect on Platelets & Coagulation Factors

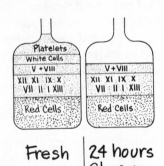

Fresh | 24 hours Storage

New platelets virtually disappear from blood after approximately 24 hours of storage. Some clotting factors also slowly lose activity on storage. The most labile is factor VIII which falls to 80% of its original value after 24 — 48 hours of storage.

"Massive Transfusion Syndrome"

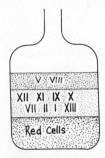

24 hours Storage.

The significance of the lack of stability of platelets, to storage in vitro is considered in more detail later. Suffice it to say here that it is obvious that if a patient is transfused with large volumes of blood which have been stored for more than 24 hours, a state of platelet depletion could be produced. This is known as "Massive Transfusion Syndrome" and may result in bleeding.

Consumption of Clotting Factors during Coagulation

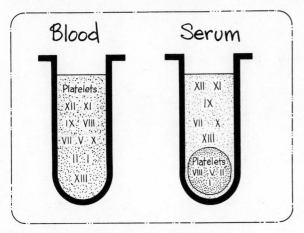

This diagram summarizes the data on consumption of clotting factors which occurs during blood coagulation. On the left are the clotting factors which are present in fresh blood and on the right the clotting factors which remain in the serum after a blood clot has formed. It can be seen that during blood clotting, platelets, factors VIII, V, II (which is prothrombin) and I (which is fibrinogen) are consumed. In addition there is partial consumption of factors XII, XI and XIII.

Consumption Coagulopathy

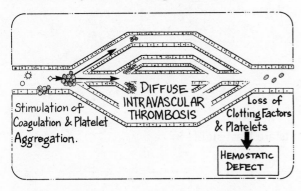

Excessive destruction of coagulation factors in vivo is seen in diffuse intravascular thrombosis in which the substrates in the clotting process are consumed as a result of widespread clotting in small blood vessels.

The resulting abnormality is known as consumption coagulopathy.

Deficiencies caused by Antibodies

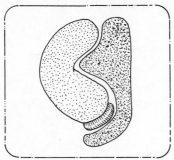

Finally, coagulation deficiencies may be caused by a specific circulating antibody to the coagulation factor. This is seen in some hemophiliacs and also in autoimmune disorders such as lupus erythematosus. These antibodies combine with and inactivate the coagulation protein, but do not lead to premature removal of the protein from the circulation.

Self Evaluation for Chapter 6

1. Which of the clotting factors are synthesized in the liver?

   1 _____   1 _____
   2 _____   2 _____
   3 _____   3 _____
   4 _____ Which are Vitamin 4 _____
   5 _____ K dependent?
   6 _____
   7 _____

2. Which of the clotting factors are consumed in blood coagulation?

   1 _____
   2 _____
   3 _____
   4 _____
   + _____

3. Which of the clotting components are least stable in stored bank blood?

4. Which of the coagulation factor deficiencies is not associated with abnormal bleeding?

5. What are possible mechanisms that produce low levels of coagulation factor activity?

Chapter 7

Inherited Coagulation Disorders

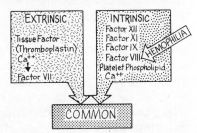

DEFECT	MODE OF INHERITANCE	INCIDENCE
XII	Autosomal Recessive	V. Rare
XI	Autosomal Recessive	Rare
IX Christmas D.	Sex linked Recessive	Uncommon
VIII Hemophilia	Sex linked Recessive	Uncommon
VIII VonWillebrands D	Autosomal Dominant	Uncommon
VII	Autosomal Recessive	Very Rare
X		
V	AUTOSOMAL RECESSIVE	VERY RARE
II (Prothrombin)		
I (Fibrinogen)		
XIII		

Hereditary deficiencies of each of the ten plasma clotting factors have been described. Not all of these inherited coagulation disorders will be considered, but rather hemophilia will be used as a model for the clinical manifestations and treatment of other inherited coagulation deficiencies. Von Willebrand's disease will also be considered because this condition has features which are not found in the other coagulation factor disorders.

Hemophilia

EXTRINSIC
Tissue Factor (Thromboplastin)
Ca⁺⁺
↓
Factor VII

INTRINSIC
Factor XII
Factor XI
Factor IX
Factor VIII — HEMOPHILIA
Platelet Phospholipid
Ca⁺⁺

COMMON

Hemophilia is due to a factor VIII abnormality and is transmitted as a sex-linked recessive trait.

Inheritance (sex-linked recessive)

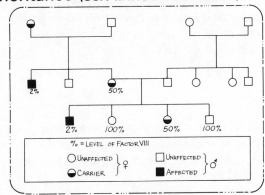

% = LEVEL OF FACTOR VIII

○ UNAFFECTED ♀
◑ CARRIER

□ UNAFFECTED ♂
■ AFFECTED

This shows the typical mode of inheritance seen in a patient with hemophilia. The clinical disorder is seen only in affected males, shown as the blocked squares. Females, on the other hand, carry the trait, but do not, except with rare exceptions, have a significant coagulation factor deficiency. Thus the affected males in this particular family had 2% of the normal coagulation factor, while the affected females had approximately 50%.

Mechanism of Factor VIII Deficiency

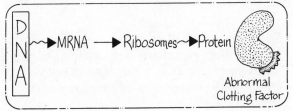

D
N
A → MRNA → Ribosomes → Protein

Abnormal Clotting Factor

The factor VIII deficiency in hemophilia as we have already mentioned results from synthesis of an abnormal molecule. This does not have biological clotting activity, but retains immunological identity with the normal factor VIII.

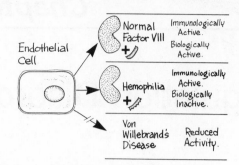

It is known that the **factor VIII** molecule is synthesized in endothelial cells in both normal people and in hemophiliacs, but in hemophiliacs it does not acquire biological clotting activity. The abnormality contrasts with the factor VIII deficiency in von Willebrand's disease in which there is a relative or absolute failure of synthesis of the molecule.

Severity

Laboratory Defect	Clinical Manifestation
<1%	Severe
1~5%	Moderate
5~20%	Mild

Various grades of severity of hemophilia are recognized and the severity of the clinical manifestations closely parallel the concentration of factor VIII in the patient's plasma. Patients with less than 1% of the factor VIII are severely affected, while those with 1% – 5% are moderately affected, and those with 5% – 20% only mildly affected.

Laboratory Defect	Clinical Manifestation	Bleeding Symptoms
<1%	Severe	Early Childhood Spontaneous
1~5%	Moderate	Usually Only After Trauma. May Be Spontaneous
5~20%	Mild	After Trauma. Local Lesions.

Bleeding manifestations in severely affected patients are usually obvious in early childhood and tend to be both severe and spontaneous. The first manifestation in patients with severe hemophilia may be bleeding following circumcision, but many severely affected hemophiliacs do not bleed abnormally until they reach the toddling stage. On the other hand, moderately affected patients do not bleed spontaneously unless they have a local lesion, for example, a peptic ulcer and these patients may have their episode of abnormal bleeding in adult life following operative trauma.

Hemophiliac Bleeding

1. SPONTANEOUS
2. POST TRAUMATIC

Both from a clinical and therapeutic point of view hemophiliac bleeding can be divided into spontaneous bleeding and post-traumatic bleeding.

Spontaneous

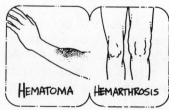

HEMATOMA   HEMARTHROSIS

Spontaneous bleeding occurs only in severe hemophiliacs and characteristically affects joints and muscles and may lead to permanent crippling unless treated promptly and adequately.

Post-traumatic Bleeding

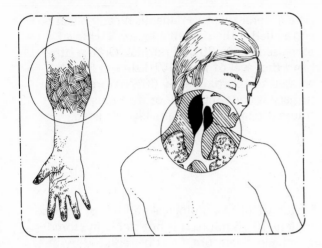

Post-traumatic bleeding characteristically occurs in deep wounds which often produce dangerous bleeding which continues for days. The large hematomas thus formed can produce pressure on nerves and occasionally even produce severe vascular occlusion leading to gangrene. Oropharyngeal bleeding is one of the most dangerous complications of hemophiliac hemorrhage because it can produce severe respiratory obstruction. This form of bleeding often follows trivial injury to the mouth and tongue.

Principles of Treatment

GENERAL:
1. Social & Psychological Care.
2. Avoidance of Injury.
3. Supportive treatment for bleeding & pre-surgery.

The general principles of treatment of any life-long bleeding abnormality are summarized here. Social and psychological care is very important. The physician must be prepared to deal not only with the episodes of bleeding, but with many of the social and psychological problems that both the patient and parents will almost invariably encounter. Whenever possible the patient should be managed in consultation with medical and para-medical specialists familiar with the problem of life-long bleeding disorders. The problem of avoiding injury is a difficult one. The parents should be encouraged to bring up their child as normally as is consistent with safety. During infancy and early childhood every attempt should be made to minimize injury by appropriate padding of cribs and by avoiding sharp toys. Later the child should be encouraged to participate in non-contact sports. When bleeding occurs the patient should be provided with supportative treatment. This includes local measures at the site of bleeding and correction of the defect by replacement therapy. Local measures should not be regarded as a substitute for replacement therapy, but merely as an adjunct because it is much more difficult to treat hemorrhage once a large hematoma has developed, than to prevent it or to treat it in the early stages.

Control of Bleeding

SPONTANEOUS—
factor VIII 20%

POST TRAUMATIC—
factor VIII 60%

As a general rule spontaneous bleeding can be controlled if the patient's factor VIII level is increased above 20% of normal. On the other hand the level of factor VIII should be increased to approximately 60% before major surgery is contemplated, or if serious post-traumatic bleeding has already occurred.

FACTOR	½ LIFE (Hours)
VII	4-5
V VIII	10-15
IX	25
X XI XII	40
II Prothrombin	60
Fibrinogen, XIII	90
Platelets	100-120

Factor VIII has a biological half-life of approximately **10-15 hours.** It is not stable in stored blood and, therefore, must be replaced by infusion of fresh blood or products prepared from fresh blood.

Factor VIII Replacement

1. Fresh Frozen Plasma.

2. Cryoprecipitate

3. Other Fractionation Procedures.

The materials available for replacing factor VIII include fresh frozen plasma which is prepared from fresh blood as soon as the blood is taken from the donor, or factor VIII concentrate, which is prepared as a cryoprecipitate or by other fractionation procedures. The factor VIII is concentrated approximately 12 fold by cryoprecipitation, but greater purity can be obtained using newer fractionation procedures.
Fresh frozen plasma is rarely used now since factor VIII levels can be more effectively raised by using factor VIII concentrates.

Effective Hemostatic Level

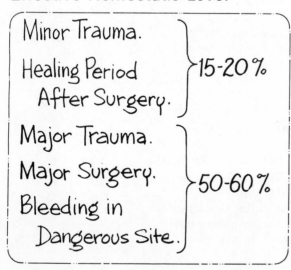

Minor Trauma.
Healing Period After Surgery. } 15-20%

Major Trauma.
Major Surgery.
Bleeding in Dangerous Site. } 50-60%

This is a list of the effective hemostatic level of factor VIII in various circumstances. The effective hemostatic level is 15% — 20% following minor trauma or following the healing period after surgery, but the level is 50% — 60% following major trauma, if major surgery is contemplated, or if there is bleeding in a dangerous site. Infusion of fresh frozen plasma is adequate to elevate the factor VIII concentration to 20% of normal, as long as the patient can tolerate the volume of fluid, but a factor VIII concentrate, such as cryoprecipitate, is necessary to elevate the level to 50% — 60% of normal.

Therapeutic Response

Severe Hemophiliac (Adult)

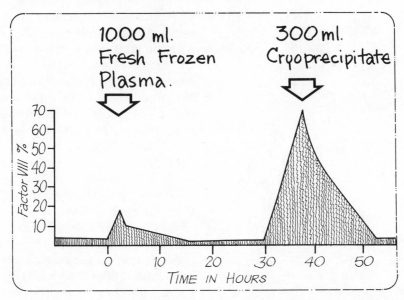

This graph shows a typical therapeutic response of a patient with severe hemophilia to fresh frozen plasma, shown on the left of the graph, and to cryoprecipitate shown on the right-hand side of the graph. Following the infusion of 1000 ml. of fresh frozen plasma to a patient with severe hemophilia, the factor VIII level rises to approximately 20% and then decays over a period of 10 hours. On the other hand, after infusion of 300 ml. of cryoprecipitate, the factor VIII level rises to over 60% and then falls to pretreatment levels in approximately 10 — 15 hours.

Local Treatment

REST
&
PROTECTION
FROM
FURTHER
TRAUMA.

The local measures used in treating hemophilia include resting the affected part and protecting it from further trauma. If the bleeding site is obscured by a large blood clot, as often occurs with mouth bleeding, and in particular after tooth extraction, the clot should be gently removed after replacement therapy has been given and a gauze soaked in a coagulant such as bovine thrombin applied to the area. Suturing of wounds should be avoided if possible, and if indicated, should only be carried out after adequate replacement therapy.

REVOLUTION

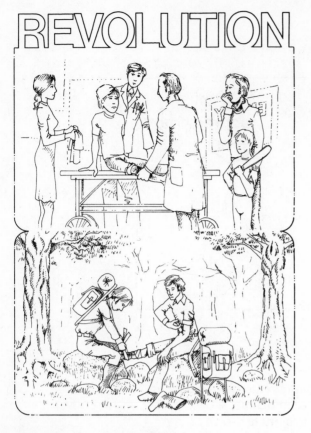

There has been a revolution in the care of hemophiliacs in recent years. This is because with the increased availability of more purified factor VIII concentrates, it is now possible to teach the hemophiliac child to treat himself at home at the earliest suspicion of a bleed. The factor VIII concentrate is stored in an ordinary refrigerator, the hemophiliac dissolves this freeze-dried concentrate, applies the tourniquet to his arm and injects the factor VIII concentrate. This approach has greatly increased the mobility of families, since the concentrate can be taken with them, when they go on vacation, for instance. It has made the hemophiliac and his family far less dependent upon the medical profession. It has virtually abolished crippling hemarthroses, and it has markedly decreased the need for hospital care.

Christmas Disease

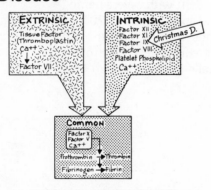

Christmas disease is due to a deficiency of Factor IX.

SEX-LINKED RECESSIVE.

FACTOR LEVELS RELATED TO SEVERITY OF DISEASE.

FACTOR IX more STABLE.

Like hemophilia it is transmitted as a sex-linked recessive trait. Similarly, there is a relationship between the levels of factor IX deficiency and the severity of bleeding. However, factor IX is much more stable in vitro and has a longer survival in the circulation.

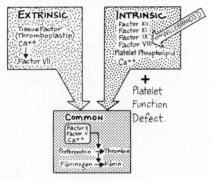

STORED
PLASMA
can be used for
replacement.

Because of its stability in vitro, stored plasma can be used for replacement therapy, and because of its longer half-life infusions do not have to be given as frequently. Recently a factor IX concentrate has been made available in Canada and the United States and this has greatly facilitated the prophylactic and therapeutic management of these patients.

Von Willebrand's Disease

The pathogenesis and classification of von Willebrand's disease has been the subject of considerable confusion. However, it is now accepted that von Willebrand's disease is a hereditary disorder, which is due to a deficiency of factor VIII and an associated platelet function defect.

Inheritance

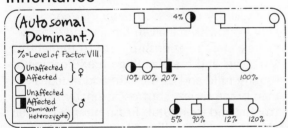

It is transmitted as an autosomal dominant trait. Thus, the disorder is transmitted from parent to child irrespective of their sex, as shown in the diagram.

Characteristics

Prolonged Bleeding
Time.

Low Factor VIII.

Defective Platelet
Function.

It is characterized by a prolonged bleeding time, a low factor VIII level and defective platelet function which is caused by the lack of a plasma factor. This platelet function defect can be demonstrated either by measuring adherence of platelets to glass beads (the glass beads retention test) or by measuring platelet aggregation induced by the antibiotic ristocetin. The platelet aggregating effect of ristocetin was a side effect which precluded its therapeutic use as an antibiotic.

Factor VIII Deficiency

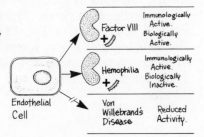

In this disorder the low biological factor VIII activity is paralleled by low immunological factor VIII reactivity suggesting that the molecule is not synthesized or is sufficiently abnormal to result in loss of immunoreactivity.

Platelet Defect

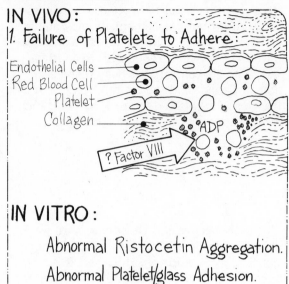

IN VIVO:

1. Failure of Platelets to Adhere

- Endothelial Cells
- Red Blood Cell
- Platelet
- Collagen

ADP

? Factor VIII

IN VITRO:

Abnormal Ristocetin Aggregation.

Abnormal Platelet/glass Adhesion.

The missing plasma factor responsible for the platelet function defect is either factor VIII itself or a molecule closely associated with it. There is evidence that this plasma factor (von Willebrand factor/factor VIII) is required for the adhesion of platelets to subendothelium, the adhesion of platelets to glass surfaces & for the aggregation of platelets with ristocetin.

The abnormal ristocetin aggregation and platelet glass adhesion are diagnostic tests which can be considered to be the in vitro counterparts of this in vivo hemostatic defect.

Severity & Treatment

- Variable.

MILD
↓
SEVERE.

- Controlled with fresh Plasma.

The severity of the disorder varies considerably even within a given family and usually bears a close relationship both to the factor VIII level and the bleeding time. Bleeding is usually mild and of the skin and mucous membrane variety, but occasionally catastrophic and even fatal. Fresh plasma is often effective in controlling bleeding. It produces an increase in factor VIII both because it contains the clotting factor and because it induces its synthesis in patients with von Willebrand's disease.

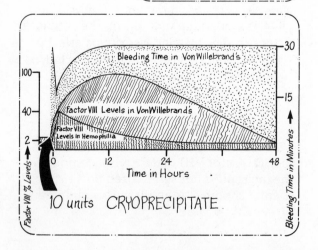

10 units CRYOPRECIPITATE.

Following transfusion, there is an immediate rise in factor VIII equivalent to the amount infused, followed by a slow rise of factor VIII which reaches a maximum in 6 – 12 hours and falls to pretreatment levels in 48 hours. The bleeding time is also sometimes shortened following transfusion of fresh plasma, but the effect only lasts for up to 3 hours after infusion.

Preparation for Surgery

SHORTEN BLEEDING TIME.

RAISE FACTOR VIII LEVEL.

When patients with von Willebrand's disease require surgery, attempts should be made to shorten the bleeding time as well as to increase the factor VIII level. This can best be done by frequent cryoprecipitate infusions (e.g. every 3 hours). If the bleeding time is not reduced, then operative bleeding may be severe despite normalization of the factor VIII level by cryoprecipitate infusions.

Self Evaluation for Chapter 7

1. How is hemophilia transmitted?

2. What are the characteristic sites of bleeding in severe hemophilia?

3. How would you define von Willebrand's disease?

4. How would the treatment of hemophilia (factor VIII deficiency) differ from the treatment of Christmas Disease (factor IX deficiency)?

Chapter 8

Acquired Coagulation Disorders

Vascular Defects.
Thrombocytopenia.
Thrombocytopathia.
COAGULATION DEFECTS.
Excessive Fibrinolysis.

The general principles of abnormal bleeding due to defective blood coagulation have already been considered. The hereditary coagulation disorders were discussed in the previous chapter. Here, the acquired coagulation disorders will be discussed.

Acquired Coagulation Disorders Associated with MULTIPLE Clotting Factor Deficiencies.

The acquired coagulation disorders are seen more commonly in clinical practice than the inherited disorders. Unlike the inherited coagulation disorders, the acquired disorders are usually associated with multiple clotting factor deficiencies. The diagnosis of the disorder is often suggested by associated clinical features and by results of screening tests, such as the prothrombin time, the thrombin time, the partial thromboplastin time and the platelet count.

Vitamin K Deficiency.
Liver Disease.
Massive Transfusion Syndrome.
Diffuse Intravascular Thrombosis.
Primary Pathological Fibrinolysis.

The following acquired coagulation disorders will be considered; Vitamin K deficiency, liver disease, massive transfusion syndrome, diffuse intravascular thrombosis, and primary pathological fibrinolysis.

Vitamin K Deficiency
Sites of Synthesis:

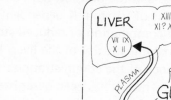

Vitamin K is required for the hepatic synthesis of factor II, VII, IX and X.

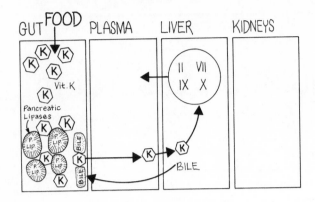

In this diagram the gut, the plasma, liver and kidneys are represented as a series of compartments. Vitamin K is obtained from food, especially green vegetables. It is a fat soluble vitamin, and therefore, is dependent on pancreatic lipases, bile and the absorptive action of the gut wall itself for its absorption into the plasma and subsequent utilization in the liver.

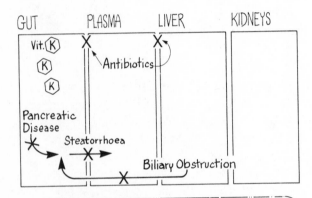

PRINCIPLES of TREATMENT.

1. Correct Causative Disorder.

2. Administration of Vitamin K.

3. Blood Transfusion for Severe Bleeding.

Vitamin K deficiency in adults usually occurs in conditions that produce fat malabsorption. This includes biliary obstruction causing a failure of secretion of bile salts, idiopathic steatorrhea, where there is a generalized malabsorption of fat and other substances, and pancreatic disease with failure to produce pancreatic lipases. In addition, Vitamin K deficiency is potentiated by the use of antibiotic drugs. The mechanism is unclear, but could be due either to interference with absorption or utilization of Vitamin K by the liver.

The principles of treatment of Vitamin K deficiency include: correction of the cause of the disorder, for example, biliary obstruction, administration of Vitamin K, and blood transfusion if bleeding is severe & dangerous, to correct both blood loss & coagulation factor deficiencies.

Hemorrhagic Disease of the Newborn

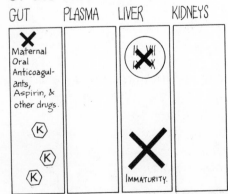

Vitamin K deficiency occurs as a different type of syndrome in the newborn. It is known as Hemorrhagic Disease of the Newborn.

This disorder, which occurs in the first few days of life is due to a defect in the synthesis of Vitamin K dependent clotting factors. It results from a combination of reduced stores of Vitamin K, and functional immaturity of the liver. It may also occur as a consequence of the administration of certain drugs to the mother. Thus, it has been described following the administration to the mother of oral anticoagulants, of anticonvulsant drugs such as phenobarbitone and phenytoin, and following the administration of large doses of aspirin.

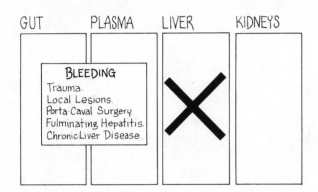

TREATMENT OF HEMORRHAGIC
DISEASE OF NEWBORN.
—Prophylactic Vit. K-1 at birth.

Hemorrhagic disease of the newborn is treated in most centres with prophylactic Vitamin K-I, given to the infant at birth.

Liver Disease

GUT   PLASMA   LIVER   KIDNEYS

BLEEDING
Trauma.
Local Lesions.
Porta-Caval Surgery.
Fulminating Hepatitis.
Chronic Liver Disease.

Some derangement of the coagulation mechanism as shown by laboratory tests, is commonly seen in liver disease. Bleeding, when it occurs, is usually only of mild or moderate degree.

Troublesome or even severe bleeding, although relatively uncommon, may occur following trauma, or if there is a local lesion, such as esophageal varices or a peptic ulcer. Severe bleeding may, however, occur when patients with cirrhosis are treated with portacaval shunt surgery or in patients with fulminating hepatitis or in patients in the terminal phase of chronic liver disease.

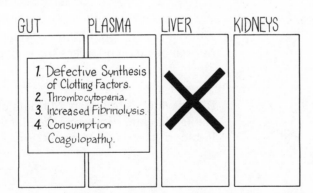

GUT   PLASMA   LIVER   KIDNEYS

1. Defective Synthesis of Clotting Factors.
2. Thrombocytopenia.
3. Increased Fibrinolysis.
4. Consumption Coagulopathy.

A number of factors may contribute to the hemostatic defect in liver disease. These include: defective synthesis of the Vitamin K dependent clotting factors that is factors II, VII, IX and X, of factor V when the liver disease is slightly more severe, and in very severe liver disease of fibrinogen. The hemostatic defect in liver disease may also be contributed to by thrombocytopenia, particularly in chronic liver disease in which portal hypertension leads to congestive splenomegaly and hence to splenic pooling. In addition increased fibrinolytic activity may occur when patients with chronic liver disease are exposed to surgery or trauma. This is because the liver is the site of synthesis of antiplasmin and the site of clearance of plasminogen activator which is released into the blood stream following surgery or trauma. The contribution of each of these factors differs depending on the associated clinical circumstances. However, defective synthesis is usually the most important factor.

Massive Transfusion Syndrome

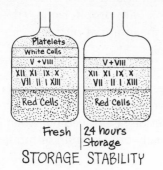

STORAGE STABILITY

Platelets are unstable in blood which is stored at 4 degrees centrigrade, that is normal bank blood.

Thus when a patient's blood volume is replaced by large volumes of stored blood, thrombocytopenia may develop because of the dilution factor.

SEVERITY OF DEFECT
- Amount of blood Transfused.
- Rate of Transfusion.
- Storage Time.
- Underlying Clinical Circumstances.

The severity of the hemostatic defect is related to several factors. These include the amount of blood transfused, its rate of transfusion, the period of time that the blood has been stored and the underlying clinical circumstances.

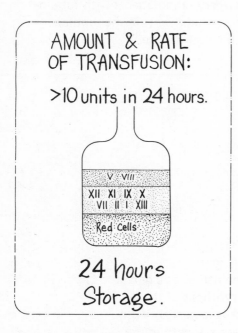

AMOUNT & RATE OF TRANSFUSION:

>10 units in 24 hours.

24 hours Storage.

Thrombocytopenia regularly occurs when more than 10 units of stored blood is administered over a 24 hour period. If the blood is given more rapidly or if larger volumes are given, abnormal bleeding or severe thrombocytopenia may occur.

Blood which is less than 24 hours old, still contains some viable platelets. However, the platelet count rapidly falls in blood stored for 24 hours or more.

UNDERLYING CLINICAL STATES

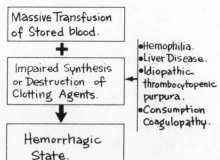

The underlying clinical state of the patient is important. The severity of the hemostatic defect produced by transfusion with large volumes of stored blood is much more marked when the capacity to produce platelets or clotting factors is impaired, for example, in hemophiliacs or in patients with liver disease. It is also more marked when the rate of consumption or destruction of platelets or clotting factors is increased, for example, in chronic idiopathic thrombocytopenic purpura or in states of consumption coagulopathy.

Management

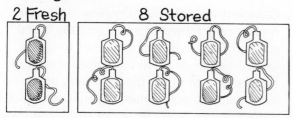

2 Fresh   8 Stored

The hemostatic defect produced by transfusion with large volumes of stored blood can be prevented or minimized if two units of fresh blood or blood which is less than 12—24 hours old is included in every 10 units of blood that is rapidly transfused.

Treatment of Established Bleeding

- Fresh whole Blood.
- Platelet Transfusion
- Fresh Frozen Plasma.

Established bleeding caused by transfusion of large volumes of stored blood is treated by administration of fresh whole blood, supplemented if necessary by platelet transfusion and fresh frozen plasma.

Consumption Coagulopathy

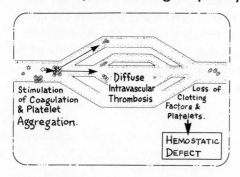

Stimulation of Coagulation & Platelet Aggregation. → Diffuse Intravascular Thrombosis → Loss of Clotting Factors & Platelets. → HEMOSTATIC DEFECT

Consumption coagulopathy is a disorder in which diffuse intravascular thrombosis causes a hemostatic defect which is due to the reduction of clotting factors & platelets as a result of their utilization or consumption in the thrombotic process. Consumption coagulopathy may complicate a variety of clinical conditions. It is usually an acute disorder, but occasionally is subacute or chronic.

Inhibitors of Intravascular Thrombosis

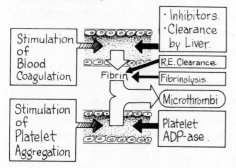

Stimulation of Blood Coagulation — Fibrin · Inhibitors. · Clearance by Liver. R.E.Clearance. Fibrinolysis. Microthrombi Stimulation of Platelet Aggregation Platelet ADP-ase.

Intravascular coagulation may be activated by relatively trivial stimuli such as mild trauma. The fact that fibrin is not continuously being laid down is due to circulating inhibitors of activated clotting factors by the liver, to the rapid clearance of small amounts of fibrin by the R.E. System, & to the fibrinolytic system.

Similarly platelet aggregation is normally prevented by the instability of platelet aggregates and by the action of plasma ADPases.

Consequently under normal circumstances significant microthrombosis does not occur.

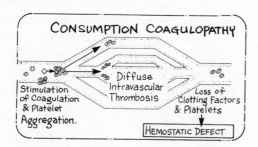

CONSUMPTION COAGULOPATHY

Stimulation of Coagulation & Platelet Aggregation. → Diffuse Intravascular Thrombosis → Loss of Clotting Factors & Platelets → HEMOSTATIC DEFECT

When extensive intravascular thrombosis does occur, however, there is a consumption of clotting factors and of platelets with a resultant bleeding tendency.

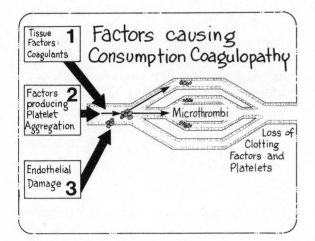

Factors causing Consumption Coagulopathy

1. Tissue Factors: Coagulants
2. Factors producing Platelet Aggregation
3. Endothelial Damage

Microthrombi

Loss of Clotting Factors and Platelets

Consumption coagulopathy may occur as a result of the release or entry into the blood stream of tissue factors which act as coagulants. In addition, it may occur as a result of factors present in the blood stream, eg. viruses, bacteria and immune complexes which induce platelet aggregation, or thirdly, it may result from extensive endothelial damage as may occur in severe trauma, burns or endotoxemia.

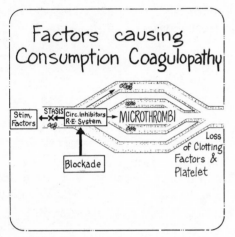

Factors causing Consumption Coagulopathy

Stim. Factors — STASIS — Circ. Inhibitors R·E· System

Blockade

MICROTHROMBI

Loss of Clotting Factors & Platelet

The condition of consumption coagulopathy is augmented by stasis, since coagulants are normally inactivated by naturally occurring circulating inhibitors, and are cleared by the liver and reticuloendothelial system, and stasis prevents the circulating inhibitors from reaching the coagulants. A consumption coagulopathy state is also augmented by blockade of the reticuloendothelial system with resulting impairment of clearance of activated clotting factors and fibrin.

Experimental Intravascular Thrombosis

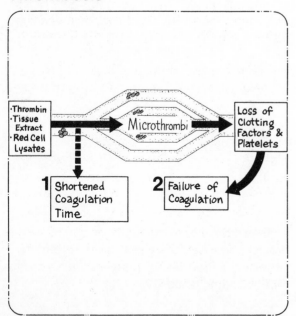

- Thrombin
- Tissue Extract
- Red Cell Lysates

Microthrombi

Loss of Clotting Factors & Platelets

1. Shortened Coagulation Time
2. Failure of Coagulation

The mechanism and consequences of consumption coagulopathy can best be understood by considering the changes which occur during the experimental induction of the process. Consumption coagulopathy can be produced experimentally by infusing thrombin, tissue extract or red cell lysates into experimental animals. These substances either initiate the clotting process, induce platelet aggregation, or do both.

The stimulation of the clotting process is first reflected by shortening of the coagulation time, but as the process continues, the blood becomes incoagulable because platelets, fibrinogen, prothrombin, and factors V and VIII are consumed during the clotting process.

Secondary Activation of Fibrinolysis

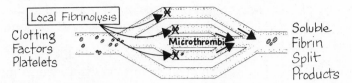

The fibrin which is formed is deposited diffusely throughout the small vessels in the body and is eventually digested by the fibrinolytic system. Widespread intravascular fibrin deposition can usually be demonstrated in animals soon after the process is induced. These deposits are no longer evident days after induction, presumably because they are digested by the fibrinolytic system which is activated as a secondary phenomenon.

The secondary increase in fibrinolytic activity is localized to the site of intravascular thrombosis and does not usually result in increased plasma or systemic fibrinolytic activity. However, the local breakdown of fibrin results in the formation of fibrin split products or fibrin degradation products which circulate in the blood stream and may contribute to the coagulation defect in consumption coagulopathy states, since these products interfere with the conversion of fibrinogen to fibrin. The significance and mechanisms of action of these fibrin split products is discussed in more detail in the next chapter.

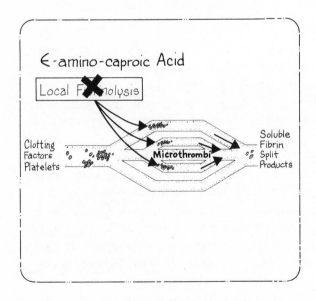

If the fibrinolytic inhibitor epsilon amino-caproic acid is given to animals early in the stages of the consumption process, widespread thrombosis with severe infarction and organ necrosis may occur, a process which resembles the "generalized Schwartzman reaction". This observation suggests that activation of the fibrinolytic mechanism which occurs as a consequence of consumption coagulopathy and diffuse intravascular thrombosis may be an important protective mechanism.

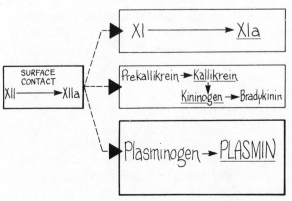

The mechanism of the secondary increase in local fibrinolytic activity is uncertain, but it may result from activation of the fibrinolytic system by activated factor XII (which is the Hageman Factor) or from the release of tissue activator from endothelial cells at the site of diffuse intravascular thrombosis, the stimulus to the release being anoxia.

Consumption Coagulopathy in Clinical Disorders

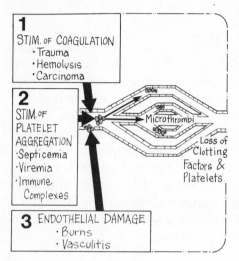

Consumption coagulopathy may complicate a number of clinical disorders. These disorders can be divided into three groups according to the principal etiological factors.

The first is stimulation of the coagulation process as a result of the release of tissue factors into the blood stream following trauma, for example, following the trauma of obstetrical accidents or surgical trauma, during acute hemolytic episodes or when there is breakdown of carcinoma tissue.

The second is induction of intravascular platelet aggregation. This occurs when the coagulation process is stimulated because thrombin causes platelets to release ADP. This also occurs in septicemia, viremia & in the presence of circulating immune complexes due to a direct effect on platelets.

The third cause of consumption coagulopathy is extensive endothelial damage which stimulates blood coagulation & platelet adhesion. Endothelial damage occurs in patients with extensive burns or in patients who have widespread vasculitis.

Clinical Manifestations of Consumption Coagulopathy

1 Asymptomatic, Abnormal Lab Tests.

2 Bleeding (Surgical Trauma, Childbirth.)

3 Organ Damage — Ischemia.

4 Microangiopathic Hemolytic Anemia.

5 Shock.

To turn now to the clinical manifestations of consumption coagulopathy or diffuse intravascular thrombosis.
In the majority of patients the process of diffuse intravascular thrombosis produces no symptoms, but evidence of consumption of platelets can be demonstrated by laboratory tests.
Bleeding may occur as a consequence of consumption of clotting factors and platelets and this is particularly severe if associated with surgical trauma or childbirth.
The third manifestation of consumption coagulopathy is organ damage due to ischemia resulting from diffuse intravascular thrombosis. The organ most severely damaged is the kidney, but there may also be organ damage to the brain or heart.
The red cells may also be damaged as they pass through the vessels, which are partly blocked by thrombus or fibrin material. This leads to marked distortion of the red cell and to a hemolytic anemia which has been called "microangiopathic hemolytic anemia".
The fifth and probably most serious consequence of consumption coagulopathy is shock. It is sometimes difficult to determine whether the shocked state is due to the underlying disorder such as septicemia, burns or trauma, due to the effects of severe blood loss, which may occur in surgical and obstetrical patients, or whether it is a complication of disseminated intravascular thrombosis.

Diagnosis

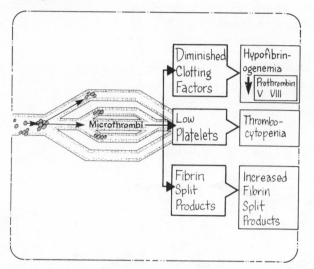

The diagnosis of the consumption coagulopathy state is confirmed by demonstrating evidence of consumption of certain clotting factors in the circulation. Thus, these patients frequently have hypofibrinogenemia, a decreased level of prothrombin, factor V, factor VIII, and thrombocytopenia. In addition there is often an increased level of circulating fibrin complexes and of circulating fibrin split products, the consequence of a local increase in fibrinolytic activity.

Screening Tests

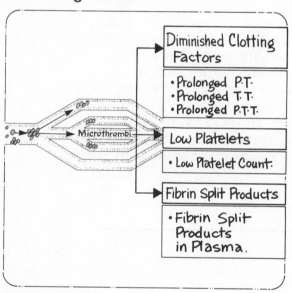

The abnormalities in clotting tests and platelets are reflected by a prolonged prothrombin time, a prolonged thrombin time, a prolonged partial thromboplastin time, by the presence of thrombocytopenia and by the presence of fibrin complexes and of fibrin split products in the circulation. It should be noted that not all of these coagulation factors which are consumed during the coagulation process are necessarily depressed in individual patients with a consumption coagulopathy state. This is because the initial concentration and rates of regeneration of these clotting factors vary from individual to individual.

Treatment

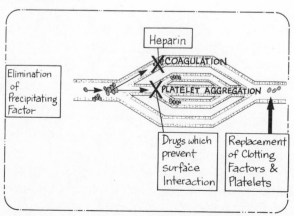

The principles of treatment of consumption coagulopathy include: elimination of the precipitating factor, for example septicemia by antibiotic treatment, replacement of the depleted coagulation factors and platelets, and inhibition of the coagulation process by heparin or of the platelet adhesion aggregation reactions by drugs which interfere with such reactions. In practice drug treatment is only required in certain circumstances.

Primary Pathological Fibrinolysis

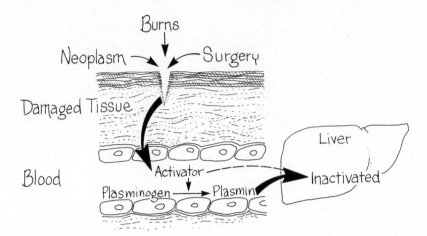

Primary pathological fibrinolysis is a hemorrhagic state which may result from a marked increase in plasma fibrinolytic activity. This is, however, a very uncommon cause of bleeding.

Primary pathological fibrinolysis may occur when large amounts of tissue plasminogen activator are released into the blood stream as a result of extensive trauma, such as may be associated with operation or breakdown of tumor tissue. Thus, bleeding due to primary pathological fibrinolysis may occur in some of the disorders which also produce diffuse intravascular thrombosis. The mechanism of bleeding and the treatment of primary pathological fibrinolysis is discussed in the next chapter.

Self Evaluation for Chapter 8

1.   List common causes of acquired coagulation disorders and the factors that are deficient in each of these disorders.

     1. _____

     2. _____

     3. _____

     4. _____

     5. _____

2.   What are the mechanisms of consumption coagulopathy?

     1. _____

     2. _____

     3. _____

3.   Why are fibrin split products elevated in patients with consumption coagulopathy?

4.   What are the causes of primary pathological fibrinolysis?

Chapter 9

Fibrinolysis

Vascular Defects.

Thrombocytopenia.

Thrombocytopathia.

Coagulation Defects.

EXCESSIVE FIBRINOLYSIS.

In this chapter bleeding disorders due to excessive fibrinolytic activity will be considered.

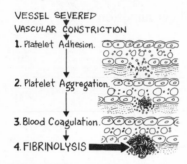

VESSEL SEVERED
VASCULAR CONSTRICTION
1. Platelet Adhesion.
2. Platelet Aggregation.
3. Blood Coagulation.
4. FIBRINOLYSIS

You will recall that fibrinolysis is the mechanism whereby a hemostatic plug or a thrombus is removed.

FIBRINOLYTIC SYSTEM

1. Physiological Fibrinolysis.
2. Pathological Fibrinolysis.
3. Impaired Fibrinolytic Activity & Thrombosis.
4. Fibrinolytic (Thrombolytic) Therapy.

The fibrinolytic system will be considered under the following headings: physiological fibrinolysis, pathological fibrinolysis, impaired fibrinolytic activity and its possible contribution to a thrombotic state, and fibrinolytic or thrombolytic therapy.

Physiological Fibrinolysis

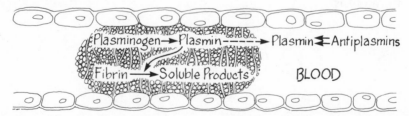

Plasminogen→Plasmin------→Plasmin⇌Antiplasmins

Fibrin→Soluble Products   BLOOD

This is a scheme of physiological fibrinolysis. Plasminogen, a beta globulin, is a pro-enzyme or zymogen which normally circulates in the blood stream in the inactive form. This is converted into the active enzyme, plasmin, by plasminogen activator. Plasmin digests fibrin, which is the desired physiological effect. In addition, plasmin digests certain clotting factors, including fibrinogen, factor V and factor VIII. It also digests other proteins. Circulating plasmin is rapidly inactivated by anti-plasmins, which are present in the blood stream in about 10 times the concentration of plasminogen. This high level of antiplasmins protects the plasma clotting factors from digestion by small amounts of plasmin, that are produced during physiological fibrinolysis.

Plasminogen Activators

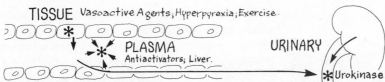

The plasminogen activators are present in tissue, in plasma, and in urine. Tissue activator is present in endothelial cells, where it exists both in a readily diffusible form, and in a particulate fraction, from where it is far less available. The endothelial activator is released into the plasma by a number of stimuli, including vasoactive agents, hyperpyrexia and exercise. The tissue activator derived from the particulate fraction of cells does not normally diffuse into the blood stream, but may become available following extensive trauma to tissues. Plasma activator is very labile, being inactivated by anti-activators which are present in the blood stream, and also it is inactivated in the liver. For this reason, enhanced fibrinolytic activity is sometimes seen in patients with chronic liver disease. The urinary activator is known as urokinase. It is antigenically distinct from tissue activator and plasma activator. Urokinase is thought to be synthesized in the kidney, and excreted in the urine. However, a small amount of the activator, which is present in the urine, does probably represent excreted plasma activator, so that there are two sources of plasminogen activator in the urine: one, an intrinsic one produced by the kidney, and two, a filtrate of plasma activator. The presence of urinary activator may be important in maintaining the patency of the renal tract.

Stimulation of Fibrinolysis

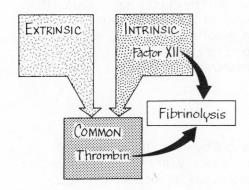

The fibrinolytic system is normally stimulated during blood coagulation. This is because activated factor XII (or Hageman Factor) accelerates the conversion of plasminogen to plasmin, and because thrombin also has a weak activating effect on plasminogen, converting it to plasmin. Thus, there is a relationship between blood coagulation and fibrinolysis; so when blood coagulation is activated, there is mild activation also of the fibrinolytic system.

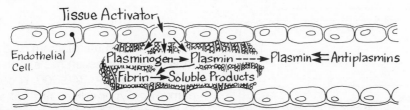

The mechanism of physiological fibrinolysis is summarized in this diagram. When a thrombus forms, plasminogen is trapped in the thrombus with the fibrin. Through unresolved mechanisms the thrombus induces the endothelial cells to release diffusible tissue activator which converts plasminogen to plasmin, close to its substrate fibrin. The fibrin is then hydrolyzed into soluble split products and the thrombus undergoes dissolution. Any plasmin that escapes from the thrombus into the blood stream is rapidly inactivated by antiplasmins which, therefore, protect the circulating coagulation factors from digestion by plasmin.

Pathological Fibrinolysis

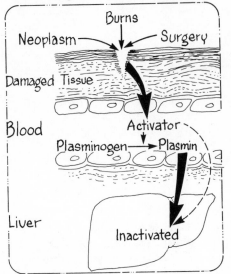

In certain conditions, known as pathological fibrinolytic states, large concentrations of plasminogen activator are released into the blood stream and may induce a bleeding tendency. Some of the causes of pathological fibrinolysis are shown on this diagram. Tissue activator may be released into the blood stream in large amounts, as a result of extensive tissue trauma, or in patients with neoplasms. In addition, large amounts of tissue activator may persist in the blood stream following even mild stimuli, if there is impaired inactivation of plasminogen activator as may occur in chronic liver disease. The activator converts plasminogen to plasmin, and the active enzyme plasmin then digests plasma clotting factors before it can be inactivated by anti-plasmins.

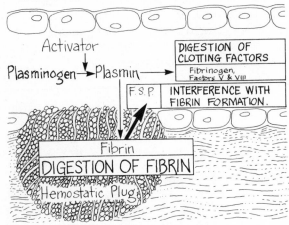

A number of factors contribute to the hemostatic defect in pathological fibrinolytic states. These include: digestion of fibrin, which is present in hemostatic plugs, interference with normal fibrin clot formation, by the presence of split products of fibrinogen or fibrin and digestion of fibrinogen, factor V and factor VIII by circulating plasmin. Of these digestion of fibrin in hemostatic plugs is the most important factor, and digestion of fibrinogen, factor V and factor VIII the least important.

Role of Products of Fibrin

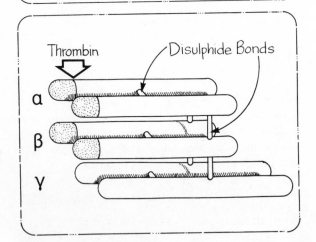

The mechanism by which the products of fibrinogen digestion with plasmin interfere with hemostasis will be considered next.

This is a schematic diagram of the fibrinogen molecule. Fibrinogen has a molecular weight of approximately 340,000. It consists of 3 pairs of polypeptide chains linked by disulphide bonds. Thrombin susceptible sites are present on the terminal portions of the alpha and beta chains. Thrombin hydrolyzes the argenyl glycine bonds, converting the fibrinogen molecule into fibrin monomer and releasing fibrinopeptides A and B into the circulation.

The three steps in the conversion of fibrinogen to insoluble fibrin are illustrated:

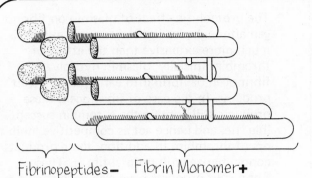

Fibrinopeptides– Fibrin Monomer+

1 The first step is a limited proteolysis of fibrinogen by thrombin to form a fibrin monomer and the fibrinopeptides.

Fibrin Polymer

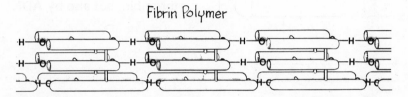

2 When the strongly electro-negative fibrinopeptides are cleaved from fibrinogen, fibrin monomer undergoes spontaneous polymerization to form a fibrin polymer. Initially, this is linked by hydrogen bonds,

Thrombin, Factor XIII, Ca++

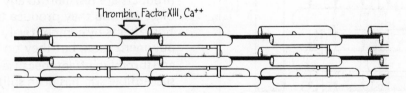

3 but in step III, the fibrin polymer is stabilized by covalent bonds. This step requires factor XIII, thrombin, and calcium.

Early Plasmin Split Products

Thrombin (at argenyl glycine bond)

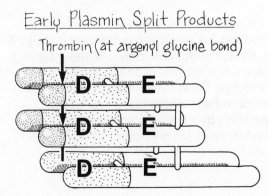

The products of limited proteolysis by thrombin should be compared with the more complete proteolysis that is produced when either fibrinogen or fibrin are digested by plasmin. The fibrinogen molecule is represented by its 2 antigenic determinants, designated D and E. Thrombin acts only on the terminal argenyl glycine bond, and this is shown by a line going through the fibrinogen molecule.

The molecular weight of the D determinant is approximately 90,000 and of the E antigenic determinant, approximately 30,000.

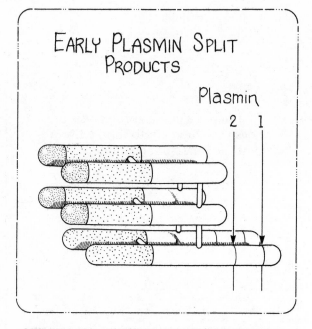

Early Plasmin Split Products

Plasmin

2 1

The proteolytic effect of plasmin on fibrinogen although also limited to some extent, is much more extensive than the effect of thrombin. Initially, plasmin hydrolyzes fibrinogen or fibrin into early plasmin split products. In the case of fibrinogen, these products still contain the thrombin susceptible site, and hence act as competitive inhibitors of thrombin. In addition, these products copolymerize with normal fibrin. These fibrin split products have also been shown to inhibit platelet aggregation, particularly by thrombin, but also by ADP.

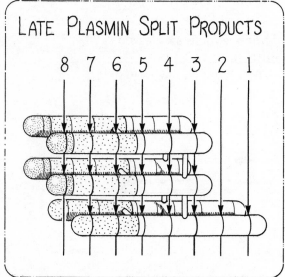

Late Plasmin Split Products

8 7 6 5 4 3 2 1

With further digestion, plasmin hydrolyzes fibrinogen into its terminal breakdown products. These late or terminal plasmin split products are resistant to any further plasmin digestion and they produce their anti-coagulation effects by competitively inhibiting fibrin polymerization, but they no longer have an antithrombin effect, because the thrombin susceptible site has been split from the fibrinogen molecule.

Summary:

Early Plasmin Split Products	• Antithrombins. • Inhibit Fibrin Polymerization. • Inhibit Platelet Aggregation.
Late Plasmin Split Products	• Inhibit Fibrin Polymerization.

In summary then, the early plasmin split products act as antithrombins, inhibit fibrin polymerization, and inhibit platelet aggregation, while the late products act only by inhibiting fibrin polymerization. The fibrin split products which result from fibrin digestion by plasmin also have a similar inhibitory effect on fibrin polymerization.

Impaired Fibrinolysis

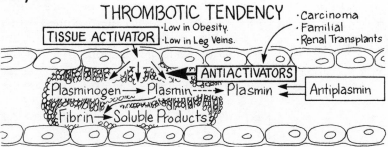

One might suppose that impaired fibrinolysis would result in a susceptibility of patients to thrombosis. The large majority of patients who develop thrombosis have no demonstrable impairment of fibrinolytic activity. However, high levels of anti-activators and anti-plasmins have been described in a small percentage of patients with a thrombotic tendency. In some cases, this has been familial, but in others it has occurred as an isolated defect. In addition, high levels of anti-activators have been described in patients with carcinoma, and in some patients following renal transplantation, particularly if the kidney is being rejected. This may be of some significance since thrombosis is a recognized complication of carcinoma and since small vessel thrombosis has been shown to occur during the renal rejection phenomenon. Low levels of fibrinolytic activity due to poor release of activator have also been described in obesity. Again, this may be of some importance since it is known that obese individuals are more susceptible to post operative and post partum thrombosis than their non-obese counterparts. Finally it has been shown that leg veins have less available activator than upper limb veins. It has also been shown that the release of activator from leg veins is impaired in some patients who develop post-operative thrombosis. This work requires confirmation, but if it is confirmed, it may be an important contributing factor to the development of venous thrombosis in the post operative period.

Fibrinolytic Therapy

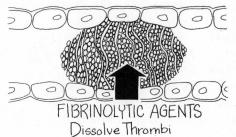

FIBRINOLYTIC AGENTS
Dissolve Thrombi

A number of fibrinolytic enzymes have now been purified, and have been used in the treatment of thrombosis. This form of treatment is known as fibrinolytic or thrombolytic therapy. There is now good experimental and clinical evidence that fibrinolytic agents can produce dissolution of thrombi in veins and arteries, and dissolution of pulmonary emboli.

Streptokinase & Urokinase

1. Activators : Streptokinase & Urokinase.
2. Streptokinase cheaper but Antigenic.
3. Urokinase Scarce but non-antigenic.

To date, the most effective thrombolytic agents have been the plasminogen activators, streptokinase and urokinase. Streptokinase is prepared from cell-free-filtrates of streptococci, but it is antigenic to man. Urokinase is prepared from human urine and has the advantage of not being antigenic to man, but urokinase is relatively unavailable and at present it is quite expensive.

Most of the early clinical experience with plasminogen activators was obtained with streptokinase, which is now available in a highly purified form, and which no longer produces the troublesome allergic reactions, that plagued the earlier preparations of streptokinase. Nevertheless the purified streptokinase is antigenic & therefore the dose used has to be tailored to the individual's needs. More recently extensive clinical experience has been obtained with urokinase as well.

Thrombolytic Therapy

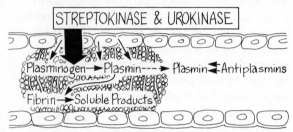

The aim of thrombolytic therapy with either streptokinase or urokinase is to deliver the plasminogen activator into the blood stream where it diffuses into the thrombus and converts plasminogen to plasmin, and hence produces dissolution of the thrombus.

Contraindications to Fibrinolytic Therapy

1. Local bleeding site, eg.- Recent Surgery.
   Peptic Ulcer.
2. Generalised bleeding Tendency.
3. Cerebro-vascular Thrombosis.

As might be expected from the foregoing discussion, the major complication of thrombolytic therapy is bleeding. Local bleeding may occur in patients who have undergone recent surgery, or in patients who have a local lesion, such as a peptic ulcer, because fibrin in the wound, or in the hemostatic plugs, is dissolved by the fibrinolytic agent. Fibrinolytic therapy is also contraindicated in patients with a generalized bleeding tendency, such as thrombocytopenia, or patients with a generalized coagulation defect, because the fibrinolytic effects would tend to augment the hemostatic defect. Finally thrombolytic therapy is contraindicated in cerebrovascular thrombosis, because so often cerebrovascular thrombosis is associated with a hemorrhagic infarct and treatment with fibrinolytic agents may produce further hemorrhage into the area of infarction.

Self Evaluation for Chapter 9

1. What are the sources of plasminogen activator?

   1 _____

   2 _____

   3 _____

2. What are the factors that contribute to the hemostatic defect in pathological fibrinolytic states?

   1 _____

   2 _____

   3 _____

3. How do fibrin split products interfere with hemostasis?

   Early   1 _____

            2 _____

            3 _____

   Late   _____

4. What are the fibrinolytic enzymes used therapeutically?

   1 _____

   2 _____

Chapter 10

Pathogenesis of Thrombosis

Hemostasis & Thrombosis

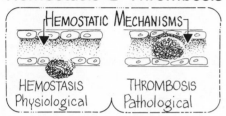

Hemostasis and thrombosis can be considered to represent two ends of a spectrum, one physiological and the other pathological. Both proceed through similar pathways, one resulting in hemostatic plug formation and the other in an occluding thrombus.

Hemostatic Mechanism

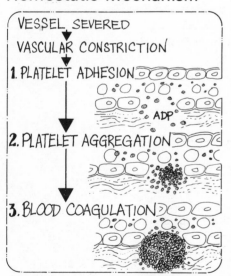

The hemostatic mechanism has already been discussed in earlier chapters. In brief, when a vessel is damaged the formed elements of the blood and the plasma coagulation factors come into contact with collagen and other extravascular tissues and initiate hemostatic plug formation.

Platelets adhere to collagen and other structures in the vessel wall, release various components including adenosine diphosphate, and platelet aggregation is induced by the released adenosine diphosphate. Activation of the blood coagulation mechanism occurs simultaneously with these platelet reactions.

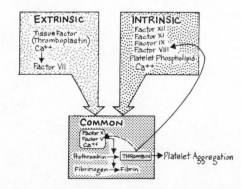

The intrinsic pathway is activated by contact of Factor XII with collagen and skin, and the extrinsic pathway is activated by tissue thromboplastin which is derived from damaged endothelial cells and fibroblasts. The blood coagulation mechanism is facilitated by the presence of platelet phospholipid also known as platelet factor III, which is made available on the surface of the platelet aggregates. Activation of the intrinsic and extrinsic pathways leads to the formation of thrombin which induces the further release of ADP from platelets and converts fibrinogen to fibrin. Fibrin stabilizes the platelet aggregates which are initially unstable and readily disrupted by intravascular pressure.

Differences between Hemostasis & Thrombosis

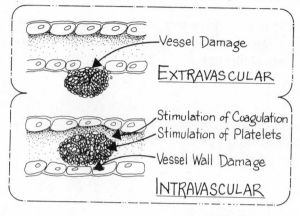

Vessel Damage

EXTRAVASCULAR

Stimulation of Coagulation
Stimulation of Platelets
Vessel Wall Damage

INTRAVASCULAR

The development and structure of the thrombus has many similarities with that of the hemostatic plug, but important differences also exist. Thus, the hemostatic plug is largely extravascular and the thrombus is intravascular. Hemostatic plug formation is always initiated by vessel damage, whereas the initiating stimulus to thrombosis may involve damage to the vessel wall, stimulation of platelet adhesion or aggregation, or activation of blood coagulation.

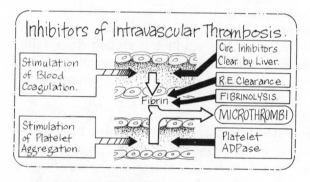

Inhibitors of Intravascular Thrombosis.

Stimulation of Blood Coagulation.

Circ. Inhibitors Clear. by Liver.
R.E. Clearance.
FIBRINOLYSIS.
MICROTHROMBI
Platelet ADPase

Fibrin

Stimulation of Platelet Aggregation.

Finally, there are a number of important protective mechanisms which operate to prevent the formation of intravascular thrombi and to check their growth.

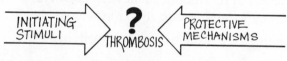

INITIATING STIMULI

? THROMBOSIS

PROTECTIVE MECHANISMS

Clinically significant thrombosis represents a breakdown in the balance between the initiating stimuli and protective mechanisms.

General Characteristics of Thrombi

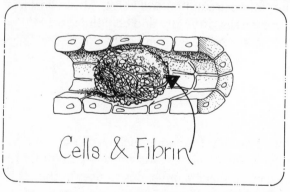

Cells & Fibrin

A thrombus is an intravascular deposit composed of fibrin and the formed blood cellular elements. The relative proportion of the formed blood elements in thrombi differs from that in blood because their accumulation is partly selective. In addition, the relative proportion of the cells to each other and to fibrin is influenced by hemodynamic factors, and therefore, the relative proportion is different in arterial and in venous thrombi.

Thrombosis in High-Flow Systems

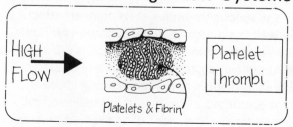

HIGH FLOW

Platelet Thrombi

Platelets & Fibrin

Thus, thrombi which form in high flow systems are mainly composed of platelet aggregates which are held together by strands of fibrin and are known as platelet thrombi.

Thrombosis & Stasis

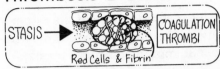

Thrombi which form in areas of complete stasis are composed of red cells with a large amount of interspersed fibrin and are known as coagulation thrombi.

Thrombosis in Moderate Flow Vessels

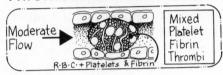

Thrombi which form in regions of slow to moderate flow are composed of a mixture of red cells, platelets and fibrin and are known as mixed platelet fibrin thrombi.

Fate of Thrombi

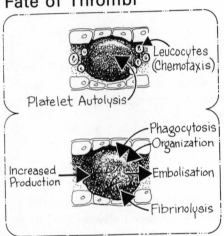

Thrombi undergo constant structual change as they age. Leukocytes are attracted by chemotactic factors released from aggregated platelets and rapidly accumulate around the platelet aggregate. In addition the aggregated platelets swell and undergo autolysis, so that after 24 hours only the fibrin remains.

The subsequent fate of the thrombus represents a balance between forces leading to deposition and removal of thrombotic material. The factors leading to removal include fibrinolysis, embolization of thrombotic material, phagocytosis of fibrin, by leukocytes, and organization of the thrombus.

Thrombus Formation at Different Sites

VEINS
ARTERIES
MICROCIRCULATION
HEART

There are four major sites of thrombus formation. These are the veins, arteries, microcirculation and heart. Although similarities exist, pathogenesis, structure and complications of these thrombi at these sites have a number of important differences.

Venous Thrombi

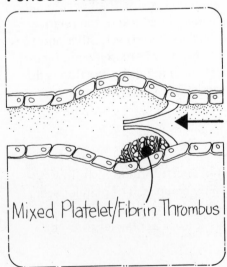

Venous thrombi are usually formed in regions of slow or disturbed flow and begin as small deposits which are commonly found in the valve cusp pockets or venous sinuses in the deep veins of the leg. These thrombi are almost always attached to the apex of the pocket, but not to the valve cusp.

The structure of the venous thrombus at its point of attachment to the vein wall is a subject of some controversy. Some investigators have reported that the initial deposits are composed of masses of platelet aggregates at their site of attachment, while other investigators have reported that these initial deposits are composed of fibrin with interspersed red cells and with only a small component of aggregated platelets.

Propagation

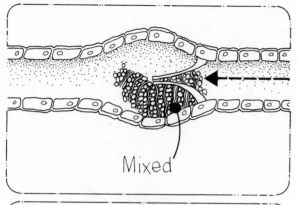

Mixed

In the initial stages of propagation the nidus grows out of the valve pocket in the direction of flow and is composed of a mixed platelet/fibrin thrombus.

When the growing thrombus starts to occlude the lumen, flow is slowed and the thrombus propagates both proximally and distally, but again mainly in the direction of flow.

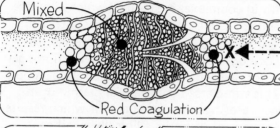

Mixed

Red Coagulation

When the lumen is totally occluded, blood flow ceases and further propagation occurs in the form of a red coagulation thrombus composed of red cells with interspersed fibrin.

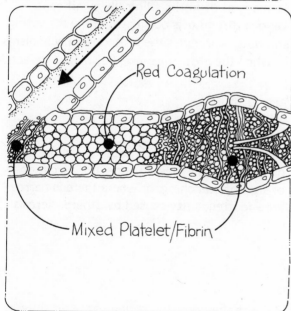

Red Coagulation

Mixed Platelet/Fibrin

Propagation continues in both directions until the next tributary is reached. This diagram of a venous thrombus shows alternating areas of a mixed thrombus and a red coagulation thrombus. When the next tributary is reached, the propagating thrombus is exposed to flowing blood and extends into the lumen as a mixed platelet/fibrin thrombus which it progressively occludes, and so the process of thrombus growth continues with alternating columns of red coagulation thrombus and pink mixed platelet/fibrin thrombus.

^{125}I-Fibrinogen Leg Scanning

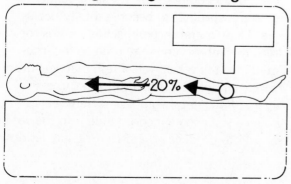

20%

Recent studies using ^{125}I-fibrinogen leg scanning indicate that venous thrombosis is a very common event in hospitalized patients who are confined to bed, but that the majority of these thrombi remain small and localized. Approximately 20% of these thrombi, however, do propagate into the large deep veins and they can lead to serious complications of pulmonary embolism and postphlebitic syndrome.

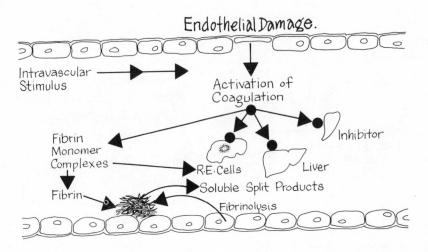

Endothelial Damage.

Intravascular Stimulus

Activation of Coagulation

Fibrin Monomer Complexes

R.E. Cells

Liver

Inhibitor

Fibrin

Soluble Split Products

Fibrinolysis

As mentioned earlier it is likely that activation of blood coagulation occurs frequently during the ordinary course of events. However, thrombosis is prevented by a well organized sequence of protective mechanisms. Thus, activated clotting factors are neutralized by their specific circulating inhibitors. If this mechanism fails due to relatively intense stimulation, activated clotting factors circulate and are cleared by the liver and reticuloendothelial tissues. Should that mechanism fail or be overcome,

fibrin complexes are formed which circulate and are cleared by the reticuloendothelial system. Once the ratio fibrin monomer to fibrinogen exceeds a critical level a fibrin gel is formed which becomes a mural thrombus. This stimulates the release of plasminogen activator from endothelial cells which results in the lysis of fibrin. Clinically significant venous thrombosis occurs when the activating stimulus overcomes the protective mechanisms or when the protective mechanisms are defective.

Arterial Thrombosis

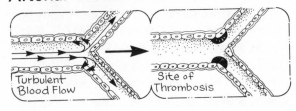

Turbulent Blood Flow

Site of Thrombosis

Arterial thrombi tend to occur in regions of disturbed flow. These may be at bifurcations or sites of branching, or where there is narrowing and irregularity caused by atherosclerosis.

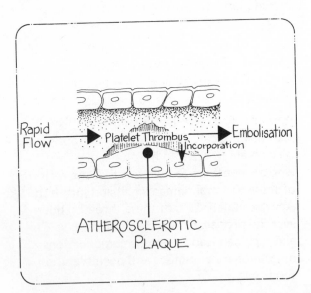

Rapid Flow

Platelet Thrombus

Incorporation

Embolisation

ATHEROSCLEROTIC PLAQUE

Because they occur in regions of rapid flow, arterial thrombi tend to remain as mural thrombi and do not have the same tendency as venous thrombi to become totally occlusive. These mural thrombi act as a nidus for fresh thrombosis and may become incorporated into the vessel wall. Fresh platelet thrombi may embolize or grow to form successive layers of platelet thrombi of different ages which also become incorporated into the vessel wall to produce atherosclerotic-like lesions.

Atherosclerosis &
Arterial Thrombosis

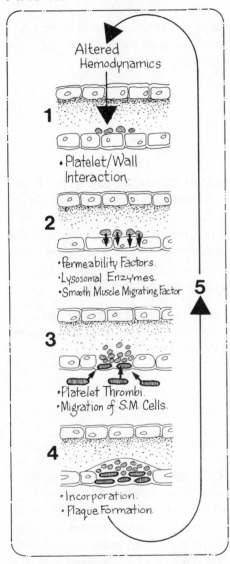

1
• Platelet/Wall
  Interaction.

2
• Permeability Factors.
• Lysosomal Enzymes.
• Smooth Muscle Migrating Factor

3
• Platelet Thrombi.
• Migration of S.M. Cells.

4
• Incorporation.
• Plaque Formation.

Altered
Hemodynamics

5

There is now considerable evidence that alterations in the hemodynamics of blood flow contribute to the development of atherosclerosis as well as to arterial thrombosis. Atherosclerotic lesions occur predominantly in regions of disturbed flow.

It has been suggested that platelets interact with the vessel wall at these sites and release permeability increasing factors and lysosomal enzymes which damage the endothelium.

In addition it has recently been shown that platelets release a substance which stimulates the migration of smooth muscle cells from the media into the subendothelial layer and this results in the formation of a plaque composed of smooth muscle cells.

Platelet thrombi may then be deposited at these sites of plaque formation or endothelial damage and become incorporated into the vessel wall. Support for this hypothesis has been provided by recent studies which have demonstrated that experimental atherosclerotic lesions can be produced by repeated endothelial injury. Thus, it is possible that the interaction of platelets and other formed blood elements with the vessel wall at sites of disturbed flow produce endothelial damage which leads to mural thrombosis and ultimately to the formation of atherosclerotic plaques. These plaques increase the disturbance of flow which may predispose to further development of mural thrombosis and hence to the growth of the atherosclerotic plaque.

Thrombosis of the Microcirculation

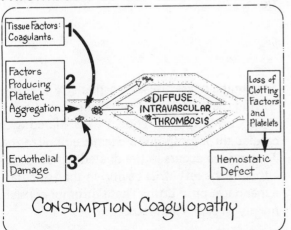

Tissue Factors: Coagulants. 1

Factors Producing Platelet Aggregation 2

Endothelial Damage 3

DIFFUSE INTRAVASCULAR THROMBOSIS

Loss of Clotting Factors and Platelets

Hemostatic Defect

CONSUMPTION Coagulopathy

Disseminated thrombosis of the microcirculation can be caused by activation of blood coagulation, by endothelial damage or possibly also by disseminated platelet aggregation. Most microcirculatory thrombi are of the mixed type containing fibrin and platelets, but in certain conditions, such as thrombotic thrombocytopenic purpura, the microcirculatory thrombi are almost entirely composed of disseminated platelet aggregates.

Cardiac Thromboembolism

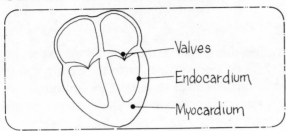

Valves
Endocardium
Myocardium

Thrombosis of the cardiac chambers occurs in disorders of the endocardium, myocardium or valve structures.

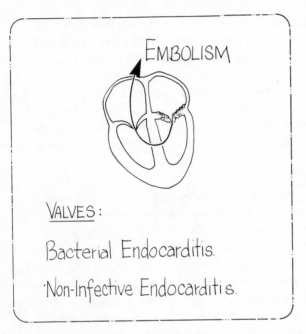

EMBOLISM

VALVES:

Bacterial Endocarditis.

Non-Infective Endocarditis.

Inflammation of the cardiac valves occurs in bacterial endocarditis and in non-infective endocarditis and is frequently associated with deposits of thrombotic material overlying the sites of endocarditis. These thrombi are usually small and consist of masses of agglutinated platelets capped with fibrin.

Embolism is fairly common and in some cases the emboli are large enough to produce serious organ infarction.

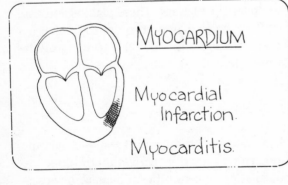

MYOCARDIUM

Myocardial Infarction.

Myocarditis.

Myocardial damage, caused either by myocardial infarction or myocarditis, can lead to areas of endocardial damage and mural thrombosis. Cardiac thrombi vary in size and consist of fibrin enmeshed in ventricular trabeculations. They may give rise to emboli which can enter the systemic or pulmonary circulations.

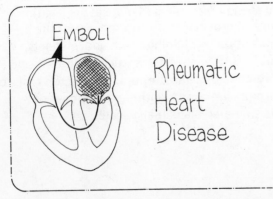

EMBOLI

Rheumatic Heart Disease

Rheumatic heart disease, particularly that involving the mitral valve and complicated by atrial fibrillation, is frequently associated with cardiac thrombosis and systemic embolization. Thrombosis occurs in the dilated left atrium either in the left atrial cavity, in the auricular appendage, or in both. These thrombi consist mainly of fibrin and red cells.

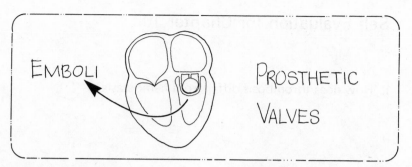

EMBOLI   PROSTHETIC
                VALVES

Thromboembolism is a well recognized complication which appears to be diminishing with the development of newer cloth covered prostheses. The thrombi are usually red thrombi consisting of fibrin, red cells with a minor platelet component. They frequently embolize and are still the commonest cause of morbidity in patients who have a prosthetic valve replacement.

Self Evaluation for Chapter 10

1. How does thrombosis differ from hemostasis?

2. What are the initiating factors in thrombosis?

3. What are the processes that protect against thrombosis?

4. How do venous thrombi differ from arterial thrombi?

5. What are the trigger mechanisms for disseminated intravascular thrombosis?

Chapter 11

Treatment of Thrombosis

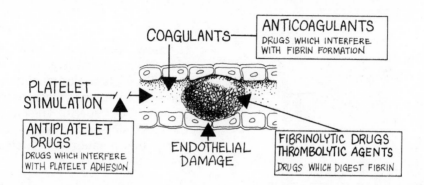

Considering the pathogenesis of thrombosis, it follows that effective prevention and treatment of thrombosis might be obtained by drugs which inhibit fibrin formation (these drugs are known as anticoagulants), by drugs which interfere with platelet adhesion and aggregation, or by drugs which digest fibrin, (these are known as fibrinolytic or thrombolytic agents). Anticoagulant drugs have been used clinically for approximately 30 years and have an established place in the treatment of venous thromboembolic disease.

Their value in arterial thrombosis is far less well established. Drugs which interfere with platelet adhesion and aggregation have been shown to prevent thrombosis in experimental animals and recent studies have also indicated that they are effective in the management of certain thromboembolic disorders in man. The fibrinolytic agents have been shown to produce dissolution of venous and arterial thrombi in man and their role in the treatment of human thromboembolic disease has recently been clarified.

The Anticoagulant Drugs

ANTICOAGULANTS
- HEPARIN
- Vit. K ANTAGONISTS

The anticoagulant drugs in clinical use are heparin and the vitamin K antagonists.

HEPARIN
- M.W. 6,000~25,000
- Immediate Effect.
- Must be given by Injection.
- Effective in Experimental & Clinical Venous Thrombosis.
- ½ Life = One hour.

Heparin is a negatively charged sulphated mucopolysaccharide with a molecular weight between 6,000 and 25,000. It has an immediate anticoagulant effect.
It is not absorbed from the gastrointestinal tract and must, therefore, be given by injection. Heparin has been shown to be effective in the prevention of venous thrombosis and pulmonary embolism both at an experimental and clinical level. Heparin has a biological half-life in man of approximately 1 hour.

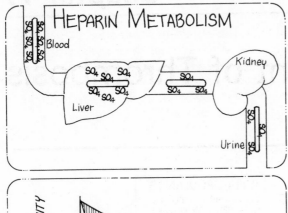

HEPARIN METABOLISM

Heparin is inactivated in the liver by removal of some of the sulphate groups and excreted in the urine in a less active form.

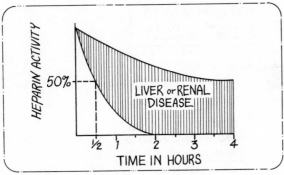

It follows, therefore, that the half life of heparin would be increased in patients with either liver disease or renal disease. The lower curve here indicates the normal rate of inactivation of heparin. The upper curve shows the much slower inactivation rate in patients with either renal or liver disease.

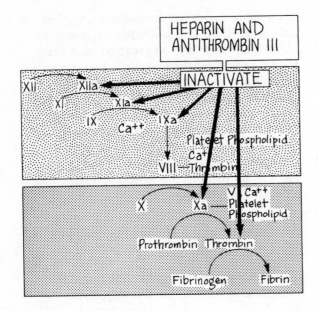

It has long been known that heparin does not inhibit the action of thrombin on purified fibrinogen, but that it requires a plasma cofactor (known as antithrombin III) for its anticoagulant effect. The interaction between heparin, the plasma cofactor and the coagulation system has recently been clarified. Heparin acts by markedly accelerating the rate of inactivation of a number of activated clotting factors including thrombin, activated factor X, activated factor IX, activated factor XI and activated factor XII by an alpha 2 globulin known as antithrombin III.

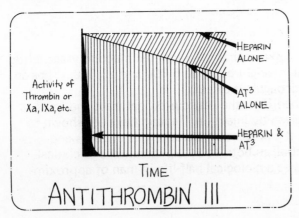

Heparin is ineffective in the absence of antithrombin III. Antithrombin III by itself irreversibly combines with a number of activated clotting factors and slowly and progressively inactivates them. Heparin, however, specifically and markedly accelerates the rate of formation of the complex between antithrombin III and the activated clotting factor, and results in immediate inactivation.

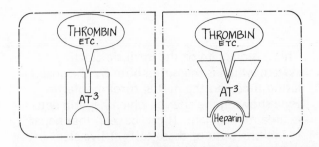

Heparin acts by binding with the antithrombin III molecule and causing a conformational change which exposes the binding site on the antithrombin III molecule for the activated clotting factor and so markedly accelerates its rate of combination with the activated clotting factor.

Administration of Heparin

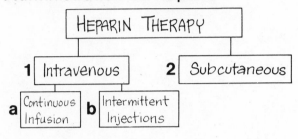

Heparin can be administered by intravenous injection either as a continuous infusion or as an intermittent injection or by the subcutaneous route. It should not be given by intramuscular injection because of the danger of local hemorrhage.

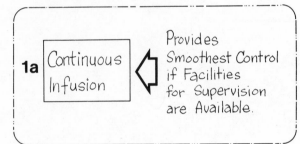

Of the three acceptable methods of administering heparin, that is continuous intravenous, intermittent intravenous and intermittent subcutaneous, the continuous intravenous method provides the smoothest control, but this method should only be used if facilities are available for careful monitoring.

Response Variance to Standard Heparin Dose

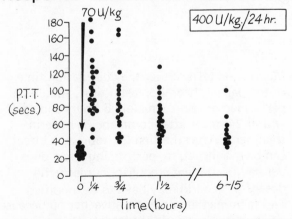

The optimal dose of heparin varies considerably from patient to patient. The diagram shows the variations in heparin level produced in 20 patients with venous thromboembolism following a standard bolus dose injection of heparin. It can be seen that the response varies considerably from patient to patient and, for this reason, the effect of heparin in each individual patient should be monitored by tests of coagulation.

Experience in animals and man has shown that a clinically significant effect can be achieved by maintaining the coagulation time at approximately 2 - 3 times the normal level at all times or the partial thromboplastin time, which is a more accurate test, at between 1½ - 2½ times normal level at all times.

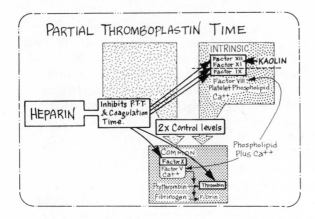

This is a diagram of the intrinsic clotting system which is measured both by the coagulation time and the partial thromboplastin time showing the sites at which heparin acts as an anticoagulant. It can be seen that heparin inhibits both of these tests at five steps in the intrinsic pathway.

Continuous Intravenous Administration

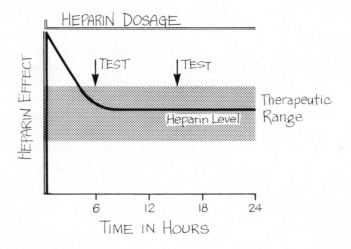

When the continuous intravenous method is used, heparin should be given as an initial loading dose of 5,000 units and then as a continuous infusion in a dose of 30,000 units administered over 24 hours. This dosage regimen will provide an adequate therapeutic level in approximately 60% of patients. In the other 40%, the dose will either have to be increased or decreased to provide a therapeutic level.

The effect of the initial loading dose of heparin and the continuous infusion can be seen in the diagram. The heparin level rises above the therapeutic range after the initial loading injection, but is then maintained in the therapeutic range during the continuous intravenous infusion.

Monitoring tests, either the coagulation time or the partial thromboplastin time, should be performed at approximately 6 hours and again within 24 hours after commencing heparin treatment. After the first 24 hours, the effect can be monitored by performing a test once per day. In patients requiring surgery, the dosage of heparin may have to be modified in the immediate postoperative period because of the danger of serious bleeding at the operative site, & also in seriously ill patients with hypotension, liver disease, or renal disease because these patients may show an increased susceptibility to the anticoagulant effect of heparin. In these circumstances, a lower dose of heparin should be used, and the effect monitored more frequently.

Intermittent Intravenous Injection

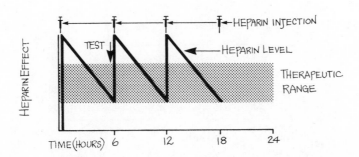

1b INTERMITTENT INJECTIONS

⬆

Fairly Smooth Control but Blood is Hypocoagulable for part of the day.

Heparin can also be given by intermittent intravenous injection, either into the side arm of a continuous intravenous infusion or as a direct intravenous injection. If the first method of heparin administration is used, heparin can be given hourly, 2 hourly or 4 hourly. However, if as is usual it is administered as a direct intravenous injection, it is usually given on a 6 to 8 hourly basis. Using this approach it is inevitable that the patient is exposed to periods of marked hypocoagulability and periods during which there is no heparin effect.

The effect of an intermittent intravenous heparin regimen, given on a 6 hourly basis, is shown here. The aim of treatment is to produce clotting tests which are in the middle to lower part of the therapeutic range before the next injection is due. To achieve this effect, it is necessary to give doses of heparin which produce levels considerably higher than the therapeutic range for 2 or

3 hours after each injection, and even then the patient is usually exposed to periods during which there is no heparin effect. When using the intermittent approach heparin is usually given in a dose of 5,000 units to 10,000 units 4 - 6 hourly, or a proportionally lower dose if the injections are given more frequently.

Subcutaneous Administration

2 SUBCUTANEOUS

⬆

Blood Hypocoagulable for Large part of the Day.

The subcutaneous route for heparin administration is particularly useful when long term treatment with heparin is indicated. However, this may lead to serious local bleeding unless special precautions are taken and again will inevitably lead to long periods of hypocoagulability, and also periods during which there is little or no heparin effect.

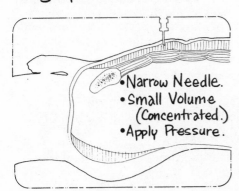

- Narrow Needle.
- Small Volume (Concentrated.)
- Apply Pressure.

The precautions that should be used to prevent local bleeding include injecting the heparin through a narrow gauge needle using a concentrated solution of heparin so that only a small volume is required and applying pressure for at least 5 minutes after injection. The most convenient site for subcutaneous heparin injection is the anterior abdominal wall. It is easy to apply pressure and there is usually a considerable amount of subcutaneous fat.

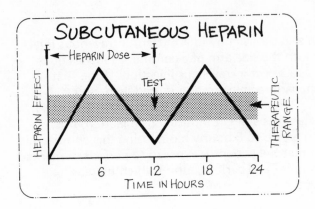

This shows the effect of 12 hourly subcutaneous heparin injections. When heparin is given 12 hourly. The normal dose is 10,000 - 15,000 u. The aim is to maintain the level of clotting tests in a therapeutic range for most of the 24 hours period. As can be seen from this diagram, this can only be achieved at the expense of having very high heparin levels for a considerable portion of the day.

Summary of Routes of Administration

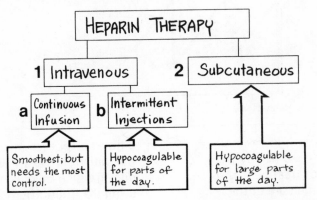

In summary then, smoothest control is obtained when heparin is given by continuous intravenous infusion, but this requires careful control, both at a clinical and laboratory level. Fairly smooth control can be obtained if heparin is given by frequent intermittent intravenous injections, but a therapeutic effect is achieved at the expense of having the blood hypocoagulable for varying periods of time throughout the day. This hypocoagulable effect is even more marked if intermittent subcutaneous heparin is used. Although these periods of marked hypocoagulability are usually well tolerated, they may be associated with an increased risk of bleeding, particularly if periods of hypocoagulability are maintained for prolonged periods of time.

Vitamin K Antagonists

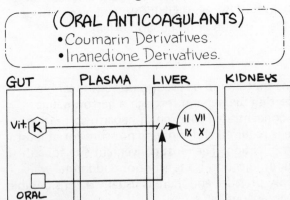

The vitamin K antagonists, which are commonly known as the oral anticoagulants, are coumarin and inanedione derivatives.

These drugs act by interfering with the hepatic synthesis of factors II which is prothrombin, VII, IX and X.

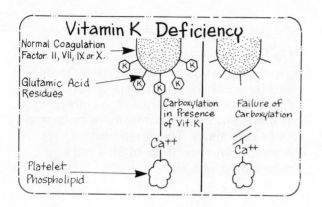

It is now known that treatment with oral anticoagulants produces abnormal II, VII, IX and X molecules. This abnormality is at a post ribosomal step in the synthesis of these protein clotting factors and the oral anti-coagulants have been shown to block car-boxylation of glutamic acid residues at one end of the clotting protein.

FACTOR	½ LIFE (HRS.)
VII	4-5
V VIII	15
IX	25
X XI XII	40
II Prothrombin	60
I Fibrinogen XIII	90
Platelets	100-120

The therapeutic effect of oral anticoagulants is delayed until the circulating clotting factors have been cleared from the circulation, this delay being 36 to 48 hours with the commonly used anticoagulants.

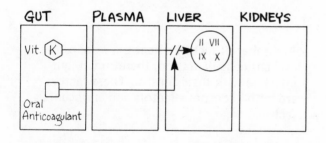

They have the advantage over heparin of being absorbed from the gastrointestinal tract, and therefore, they can be given orally, however, they are probably less effective than heparin as anti-thrombotic agents.

Commonly Used Vitamin K Antagonists & Effects

Drug	Therapeutic Effect	Length of Action	Side Effects
Warfarin	36-48 hrs.	Intermediate	Few
Phenindione	36-48 hrs.	Intermediate	more
Ethyl Biscoumacetate	18-30 hrs.	Short	Few
Phenprocoumin	48-60 hrs.	Long	Few

This shows the therapeutic effect of the four commonly used vitamin K antagonists. Of these, warfarin, a coumarin derivative, is most widely used. Both are equally effective as anticoagulants and are well absorbed. However, warfarin is the preferred agent because its use is associated with a low incidence of side effects. The serious side effects of phenindione include agranulocytosis. Both

warfarin and phenindione have an intermediate length of action and produce their therapeutic effect within 36 to 48 hours. On the other hand ethyl biscoumacetate has a shorter therapeutic effect and a shorter length of action, while phenprocoumin has a longer therapeutic effect and a longer length of action.

Monitoring

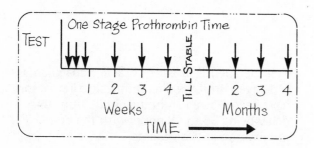

Vitamin K Antagonists

Aim to keep One stage
Prothrombin Time at 2X normal.

The effects of the oral anticoagulants on blood coagulation can be adequately monitored by either the one stage prothrombin time. The aim is to maintain the clotting time of these tests at approximately twice control levels at all times. This is represented by a prothrombin time of 15 to 30% and a thrombotest of 5 to 15%.

One Stage Prothrombin Time

TEST

TILL STABLE

1 2 3 4 | 1 2 3 4

Weeks Months

TIME ➡

Either one of these tests is performed 3 times in the first week after commencing the oral anticoagulants and then weekly until the maintenance dose is stable and then at bi-weekly or monthly intervals.

Factors Affecting Response to Oral Anticoagulants

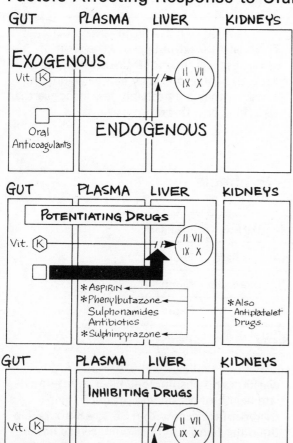

GUT   PLASMA   LIVER   KIDNEYS

EXOGENOUS

Vit. Ⓚ

II VII
IX X

Oral
Anticoagulants   ENDOGENOUS

GUT   PLASMA   LIVER   KIDNEYS

POTENTIATING DRUGS

Vit. Ⓚ

II VII
IX X

*ASPIRIN
*Phenylbutazone
Sulphonamides
Antibiotics
*Sulphinpyrazone

*Also
Antiplatelet
Drugs.

GUT   PLASMA   LIVER   KIDNEYS

INHIBITING DRUGS

Vit. Ⓚ

II VII
IX X

Barbiturates

A number of factors affect the response to oral anticoagulants and, therefore, might interfere with their control. These factors are both exogenous factors and endogenous factors.

A number of drugs, including aspirin, phenylbutazone, sulphonamides, oral antibiotics, & sulphinpyrazone augment the effect of vitamin K antagonists. These act by displacing the oral anticoagulant from its carrier protein (albumin), & hence making it more available for hepatic inhibition of vitamin K. Troublesome and even dangerous bleeding may result if they are taken by patients who are well controlled on oral anticoagulant treatment. Some of these drugs, namely aspirin, sulphinpyrazone and phenylbutazone also suppress the interaction of platelets with surfaces and may contribute to bleeding because of this effect.

Of the drugs that inhibit the vitamin K antagonists, barbiturates are the most important. These barbiturates and other sedatives may increase dosage requirements of the oral anticoagulants because they inhibit the action of vitamin K antagonists and, therefore control may be poor when the patient is discharged from hospital and stops taking the sedative.

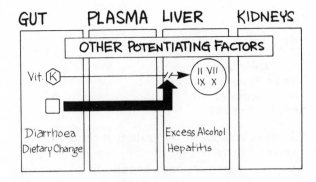

Other factors which interfere with anti-coagulant control include potentiating factors such as excessive alcohol intake, because of its interference with liver function, diarrhea, because of its interference with vitamin K absorption, a change in diet, whereby less vitamin K is present in the diet, and liver disease, such as hepatitis, because the synthesis of the vitamin K dependent clotting factors is affected by liver disease.

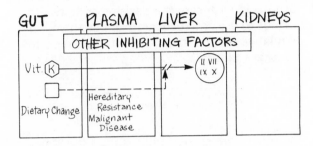

The other factors which inhibit the vitamin K antagonists include a change in diet, in which the vitamin K content of the diet is increased, malignant disease and hereditary resistance to vitamin K antagonists.

Bleeding during Anticoagulant Therapy

- Uncommon.
- Post-operative.
- Unmasked Local Lesions.

Bleeding during oral anticoagulant therapy is relatively uncommon, if the tests used to monitor therapy are maintained within the defined therapeutic range. However, there is always a danger of postoperative bleeding and the anticoagulant effect may unmask the presence of a local lesion such as a carcinoma, peptic ulcer, or renal calculus and hence produce local bleeding.

Antidotes

BLEEDING!	ANTIDOTE
Heparin	Protamine Sulfate (1mg/100u)
Vitamin K Antagonists	Vitamin K^1 (25 mg. I.V.)

Serious bleeding due to heparin therapy should be treated with the antidote protamine sulfate. This strongly basic compound combines with and inactivates heparin immediately. Approximately one mg. of protamine sulfate neutralizes approximately one mg. which is 100 units of heparin. The neutralizing dose of protamine depends both on the route of administration of heparin and the time of the last injection.

Overdose of vitamin K antagonists may be relative, due to ingestion of certain drugs which augment the effect of vitamin K, or absolute. Bleeding associated with overdose may be spontaneous and severe. When a patient being treated with the vitamin K antagonists bleeds excessively, the bleeding should be treated with vitamin K-1 given by injection in a dose of 25 mg. If it is life-threatening, the patient should be treated with II, VII, IX and X concentrate.

Contraindications to Anticoagulant Therapy

ABSOLUTE	RELATIVE
Active Peptic Ulcer	Hemostatic Defect
Completed Stroke	Severe Hypertension
	Liver Disease
	Renal Disease.

The contraindications to anticoagulant therapy include absolute contraindications, such as patients with an active peptic ulcer, because of the danger of bleeding from the ulcer or patients with a recent completed stroke because of the danger of bleeding into the area of cerebral infarction; and relative contraindications, such as the presence of a generalized hemostatic defect, the presence of severe hypertension because of the potential danger of cerebral hemorrhage, or the presence of liver or kidney disease, both conditions augmenting the anticoagulant effect of these anticoagulant agents. In each case the decision as to whether or not to use anticoagulants in patients with a relative contraindication will depend on the clinical situation.

Arvin

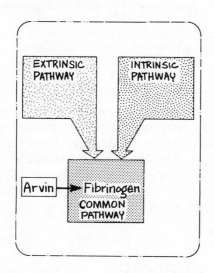

Another anticoagulant-like drug is the Malayan Pit Viper Venom, known commercially as Arvin or Ancrod. This has also been used to treat thrombosis. Arvin interacts with fibrinogen in vitro and in vivo converting it into a form of fibrin which is very rapidly lyzed by the fibrinolytic system. Preliminary studies indicate that the venom can be given intravenously or by intramuscular injection with reasonable safety in patients with thromboembolic disease. However, its therapeutic efficacy has yet to be established and there are indications that is is weakly antigenic in man.

Antiplatelet Drugs

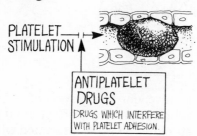

In recent years there has been considerable interest in the potential antithrombotic effect of drugs which suppress platelet function. A great many compounds have been observed to inhibit platelet function in vitro, but only a few of these agents have been shown to have antithrombotic efficacy when tested in experimental animal models in vivo and even fewer have been tested in man.

DRUGS WHICH INHIBIT PLATELET FUNCTION
- ASPIRIN.
- DIPYRIDAMOLE.
- SULPHINPYRAZONE.

Of the drugs tested in man, three have been shown to be particularly promising. These are aspirin, dipyridamole and sulphinpyrazone.

ASPIRIN	Thrombocytosis & Spontaneous Aggregation. ??? Ischemic Heart Disease
DIPYRIDAMOLE	Thrombotic complications of Heart Valve replacement.
SULPHINPYRAZONE	A-V Shunts—Chronic Renal Dialysis. ? Cerebro-Vascular Disorders. ? Recurrent Venous Thromboembolism.

The early results of studies with aspirin were inconclusive but there is now evidence that aspirin is effective in reducing the frequency of thrombosis in patients undergoing hip surgery and in reducing the frequency of thromboembolic complications in patients with transient cerebral ischemia. A number of studies with aspirin have also provided promising results in ischemic heart disease but the evidence for the effectiveness of aspirin in this condition is not yet conclusive.

Dipyridamole has been shown to be effective in preventing thromboembolic complications in patients with prosthetic heart valves.

Sulphinpyrazone has been shown to reduce occlusive events in patients with arteriovenous shunts who are having chronic hemodialysis, and there is now evidence that sulphinpyrazone reduces the frequency of sudden death in patients who are discharged from hospital with a diagnosis of acute myocardial infarction.

Fibrinolytic Agents

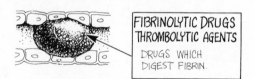

FIBRINOLYTIC DRUGS
THROMBOLYTIC AGENTS

DRUGS WHICH
DIGEST FIBRIN.

Finally fibrinolytic agents will be considered.

Streptokinase and urokinase are two fibrinolytic agents which have been shown to produce dissolution of experimental thrombi and of arterial and venous thromboemboli in man.

LYSIS OF RECENT VENOUS THROMBI { **STREPTOKINASE** } LYSIS OF PULMONARY EMBOLI

UROKINASE

Both of these drugs have been shown to accelerate lysis of major pulmonary emboli in man and have a place in the treatment of major pulmonary embolism. Streptokinase has been shown to produce lysis of recent venous thrombi in man and should be considered in young patients with extensive acute venous thrombosis. Both streptokinase and urokinase have the potential to produce serious bleeding, particularly in the postoperative period. Therefore, the decision regarding the use of these agents must always be weighed against the risks of therapy.

Indications for Anticoagulant Therapy

1. VENOUS THROMBOSIS & PULMONARY EMBOLISM.

2. PERIPHERAL ARTERIAL EMBOLISM.

3. A few special cases of Disseminated Intravascular Thrombosis.

4. ? Myocardial Infarction;
   ? Cerebrovascular disease;
   ? Arterial Thrombosis.

Finally, what are the indications for anti-coagulant drugs? Anticoagulant drugs are indicated in patients with venous thrombosis and pulmonary embolism; in patients with peripheral arterial embolism, particularly those associated with a local site for embolism such as a prosthetic heart valve; or in patients with mitral stenosis and atrial fibrillation; and these drugs are also of value in certain cases of disseminated intravascular thrombosis. The role of anticoagulant drugs in patients with acute myocardial infarction, cerebrovascular disease and arterial thrombosis is less well established.

Self Evaluation for Chapter 11

1. List the different classes of antithrombotic agents.

2. What are the respective roles of heparin and oral anti-coagulants in the treatment of venous thromboembolic disease?

3. How should heparin be administered?

4. How should heparin be monitored?

5. How should oral anticoagulants be monitored?

6. What are some of the factors which interfere with oral anticoagulant drug control?

7. What is the current status of
   a) fibrinolytic agents,
   b) anti-platelet drugs in the management of thromboembolic disease?

References

Biggs, Rosemary and MacFarlane R.G., (1972) "Human Blood Coagulation, Haemostasis and Thrombosis." Oxford, Blackwell.

Ratnoff O.D., (1960) "Bleeding Syndromes." Charles C. Thomas, Springfield, Illinois.

Williams, William J.; Beutler, Ernest; Ersler, Allan J.; and Rundles, R. Wayne; (1972) "Hematology." McGraw-Hill Book Company.

Gallus A.S., Hirsh J. "Seminars in Thrombosis and Hemostasis." Vol. II No. 4 April 1976.
1. "Diagnosis of Venous Thromboembolism."
2. "Prevention of Venous Thromboembolism."
3. "Treatment of Venous Thromboembolic Disease."